INNOVATIONS

in End-of-Life Care

Practical Strategies & International Perspectives

INNOVATIONS

in End-of-Life Care

Practical Strategies & International Perspectives

Edited by

Mildred Z. Solomon, EdD
Anna L. Romer, EdD
Karen S. Heller, PhD

Center for Applied Ethics & Professional Practice
Education Development Center, Inc.

Foreword by David E. Weissman, MD

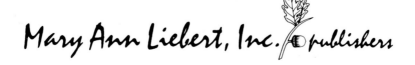

Library of Congress Cataloging-in-Publication Data

Innovations in end-of-life care: practical strategies and international perspectives /
edited by Mildred Z. Solomon, Anna L. Romer, Karen S. Heller; foreword by David E. Weissman.
     p; cm.
  Includes bibliographical references and index.
  ISBN 0-913113-87-5 (pbk.)
  1. Terminal care. I. Solomon, Mildred Z. II. Romer, Anna L. III. Heller, Karen S.
  [DNLM: 1. Terminal Care. 2. Advance Directives. 3. Dementia. 4. Pain,
Intractable--therapy. 5. Patient Care. WB 310 I58 2000]
R726.8 .I55 2000
362.1′75--dc21

                                                                          00-028735

Parts of this book appeared in a slightly different form in the electronic journal *Innovations in End-of-Life Care* **www.edc.org/lastacts**

Cover image courtesy of NASA Space Photography.

All papers, comments, opinions, findings, conclusions, or recommendations in *Innovations in End-of-Life Care* are those of the author(s), and do not constitute opinions, findings, conclusions, or recommendations of the Publisher, the Editors, and the editorial staff.

Printed in the United States of America.

Photograph Acknowledgments:

Part One p. 1. Photo by Jamie Cope ©1974. Reprinted with permission.

Part Two p. 11. Photo by Aaron Sodickson, "Doctor with Patient" ©2000. Reprinted with permission.

Part Three p. 63. Photo by John Seakwood, ©1981. From the documentary film "Walk Me to the Water," an award winning film on the special needs and insights of the dying and their families, available from Walk Me to the Water, 100 Bird Road, P.O. Box 55, New Lebanon, NY 12125, Tel. (518) 794-8081.

Part Four p. 105 Photo by Doug Mindell, "Hands Holding" ©2000. Reprinted with permission.

Part Five p. 139 Photo by Jamie Cope, ©1974. Reprinted with permission.

CONTENTS

Foreword

As someone who has been working for many years to improve palliative care in diverse health care settings, I take special pleasure in writing this foreword to *Innovations in End of Life Care: Practical Strategies and International Perspectives.* My background is medical oncology, but for the last five years I have been involved full-time in palliative care. From my point of view, one of the most helpful aspects of *Innovations* is that it provides a much broader perspective on how to make things better for dying patients and their family members than one can find anywhere else. This volume has such special relevance because it is both multi-disciplinary and multi-national. It speaks to all the health care disciplines working within hospitals, nursing homes, home health agencies, hospices, and in the community: physicians, nurses, social workers, hospital clergy, administrators, quality improvement specialists, and other allied health professionals. And it does so from an international perspective.

Readers will find this volume, an annual compendium of material that first appeared in the on-line journal of the same name, full of promising practices and helpful insights from people who have succeeded in changing practices and policies in their own institutions and communities. Each section of the book is devoted to a particular topic and features an innovative approach to improving care, as well as commentary from palliative care experts in other countries. The four topics covered in this year's collection are: truth-telling and advance care planning; family-centered care, which is about empowering patients and families to become fuller partners in setting the goals of care; cancer pain management; and improving care and maintaining connection with people with advanced dementia.

In reading these articles, I have been struck by how important it is when planning a change or an innovation to attend to the process and to the key stakeholders and their interests. One needs to involve people from all the relevant disciplines and to consider how they interact in the care of patients and what would motivate them to undertake the change. Consider the Study to Understand Prognoses and Preferences for Outcomes and Risks of Treatments (SUPPORT), for example. In that study—the largest ever in the United States to aim to improve end-of-life care—it was lack of collaboration between nurses and physicians that proved fatal to the success of the intervention.[1] The physicians never read the reports that the nurses put in the patients' charts.

There is now strong research evidence that the context in which change is attempted, and the ways in which it is introduced, are essential to the success of quality improvement efforts.[2,3,4] Through interviews with innovators in a range of settings, the editors of *Innovations in End-of-Life Care* have elicited numerous telling details about how change is actually achieved. Thus, this volume offers not only the innovators' good ideas, but also includes their personal insights about what fosters and impedes the change process.

To effect improvements in the complex arena of health care today, it is not enough to have a good idea; one has to know who the stakeholders are and what incentives will be needed to motivate all those whose help will be required to implement the change. One needs to anticipate what roadblocks might be encountered and what data and whose support would help to get traffic moving in the direction of quality improvements in care.

Recently, I had an experience that brought this home. I was asking the hospital to form a contractual relationship with a community hospice agency that I was working with, which I saw as a straightforward, somewhat bureaucratic process, because hospitals and hospices always have a contractual relationship. So, I posed this idea to the head of clinical services and nursing in my hospital, who looked me in the eye and said, "Doctor Weissman, this is an acute care hospital. Our patients do not die."

Needless to say, I was taken aback. I had not identified who the stakeholders were in the terrain in which I wanted to bring hospice and hospital together, and I had not collected the evidence to establish the need for what I was proposing. I was not prepared for her reaction nor certain about how to respond.

I went back to my office, retrenched, and began a very slow and arduous process of identifying who cared about caring for the dying. I got the people in nursing, social service, chaplaincy, and the other concerned disciplines around the table together, and we mapped out a whole series of data collection issues and educational strategies. With so many key players involved in extensive, visible activities, the hospital administration now says, "You're doing great work. How can we help you?" That experience underscored for me that one cannot sell a good idea just because one thinks it's a good idea. Potential change agents often forget that they need data and buy-in by stakeholders to move the process forward.

---

[1] The Study to Understand Prognoses and Preferences for Outcomes and Risks of Treatments (SUPPORT). A controlled trial to improve care for seriously ill hospitalized patients. *JAMA* 1995;274:1591–1597.

[2] Solomon M. The enormity of the task: SUPPORT and changing practice. In: Dying Well in the Hospital: The Lessons of SUPPORT. *Hastings Center Report (Special Supplement)* 1995;25(6):S28–S32.

[3] The University of York NHS Centre for Reviews and Dissemination. Getting evidence into practice. *Effective Health Care.* 1999;5(1):1–16.

[4] Wood M, Ferlie E, et al. Achieving clinical behavior change: A case of becoming indeterminate. *Social Science Medicine.* 1988;47(11):1729–1738.

There are many stakeholders: not only physicians, nurses and other direct providers of care, but also hospital administrators, pharmacy personnel, patients and families. Yet, too often, efforts to improve palliative care and pain management become turf battles over who is going to get to see the patients and be in charge of that aspect of their care. I hear this theme recurrently when I visit hospitals around the United States. The kinds of articles that appear in *Innovations* focus away from that kind of negative competition. Instead, these pieces demonstrate how to involve all the disciplines in improving a given aspect of palliative care within an institution, across institutions, or within a community.

This year's compendium of the best of *Innovations* online journal articles offers a rich storehouse of experience, resources, and tools in four domains of end-of-life care. Through these diverse examples, *Innovations* provides broad yet rich and detailed perspectives on how to build effective team approaches within health care institutions that want to provide humane care to the dying. You will find much to consider here, and much to inspire creative action in your own setting.

David Weissman, MD
Medical College of Wisconsin
Editor, Journal of Palliative Medicine
April 2000

Acknowledgments

Innovations in End-of-Life Care grew directly out of The Robert Wood Johnson Foundation's Last Acts initiative, conceptualized and ably led by Victoria Weisfeld, senior communications officer at The Robert Wood Johnson Foundation, Princeton, New Jersey. Thanks to Vicki's efforts and the foundation's support, there are now more than 450 Last Acts–affiliated organizations working together to improve end-of-life care. Former First Lady Rosalynn Carter serves as Honorary Chair of the campaign, which has undertaken many outstanding projects across the United States.

In 1996, Vicki invited Mildred Z. Solomon, EdD, director of the Center for Applied Ethics and Professional Practice at Education Development Center, Inc. (EDC), and Thomas Delbanco, MD, director of internal medicine at The Beth Israel Deaconess Medical Center, Boston, Massachusetts, to serve as co-chairs of one of the Last Acts' several task forces. That task force was devoted to facilitating improvements within health care institutions and it generated a number of ideas for how to help Last Acts meet its objectives. *Innovations* is the child of those first early explorations. If the truth be told, like many good ideas, it first emerged on a napkin in a coffee shop, as Vicki and Millie were discussing the problem of how to make lasting and meaningful changes within complex health care organizations. We are indebted to Vicki for her early vision of what was possible, her encouragement to use the Internet to speed the rate of innovation in end-of-life care internationally, and her continuing guidance.

The articles and interviews collected in this volume would not exist were it not for the direction and guidance we have received from our outstanding international editorial board. Its members helped us to conceptualize the themes to focus on and led us to important innovations. Although not an official member of our Editorial Board, we are most grateful to Kathleen Foley, MD, for her colleagueship on this and many other projects, as she is always generous in providing good ideas and helpful insights.

Special thanks must go to Stacy Piszcz, our competent and energetic management associate at the Center for Applied Ethics and Professional Practice at EDC. Stacy's excellent organizational skills and steady hand guided this project through many twists and turns. Our creative and efficient colleague at EDC, Elizabeth Collins, first constructed our website and managed it in its early days. Pamela Metz has served as webmaster since, ensuring that we are able to serve our online readers efficiently and post our pieces on time. We have very much appreciated Pamela's technical expertise and her willingness to work against severe deadlines. Samantha Libby Sodickson has recently joined the editorial staff of *Innovations* and serves as liaison to the publisher Mary Ann Liebert, Inc. Samantha's artistic sensibility, and familiarity with the world of publishing have smoothed the transition from manuscript to book. She designed the cover of this book and has attended to every detail in preparing this manuscript for publication.

Deborah Sellers, PhD, and Erica Jablonski assisted us with gathering user feedback through an online survey, for which we are most grateful. Judith Spross, RN, EdD, helped us develop the material on cancer pain management, presented in the editorial in Part Four of this volume. Alan Stockdale, PhD, and Sue Herz, JD, two other senior colleagues at the Center for Applied Ethics and Professional Practice, put up with our intermittent distractions and were always available for consult and moral support. Tim McIntire, our administrative assistant, willingly did research for us and assisted in numerous ways, including providing an occasional hand with transcription and editing, for which we are most grateful.

When the idea for *Innovations* was still in its infancy, Donna Williams and Julia Zauner moved the project along by providing a thorough business plan. Later, once we were up and running, Julia stayed involved and contributed by ensuring that *Innovations* was on the appropriate search engines and that we were linked with other relevant websites. The task of marketing *Innovations* online now falls to another able web marketer, Beth Brainard. Karen Long and Jill Stewart of Stewart Communications recruited the interest and support of many of the Last Acts partner organizations for the website and print versions of *Innovations*. Their efforts on behalf of this project are much appreciated.

We also wish to thank Tony Artuso, EDC's director of publishing, for his help in the ongoing revision of our business plan and for his participation and guidance as we selected a publisher. Other senior EDC staff members provided guidance and "backstopping" as we developed our ideas, including Dan Tobin, EDC's director of communications, Cheryl Vince Whitman, senior vice president, and Janet Whitla, president. We are grateful to Ellen Lubell and Amy Segal for their assistance in developing the relationship with our publisher, Mary Ann Liebert, Inc.

Indeed, we feel we have made just the right match in finding Mary Ann Liebert, Inc. We wish to thank Mary Ann Liebert and Vicki Cohn, who first had the idea of collecting the best of the Web-published material, along with new work, in an annual compendium. Larry Bernstein and Susan Jensen's conscientious efforts in the design, layout, and production of this book are greatly appreciated.

David Weissman, MD, editor-in-chief of the *Journal of Palliative Medicine*, has recently joined *Innovations* as an associate editor. We look forward to collaboration with him and *JPM*, which is now publishing excerpts from our website in each of its issues.

Finally, we want to thank our contributors for their willingness to share their work. Each contributor has been frank about the opportunities, but also the barriers, they encountered. They have been generous in their willingness to engage with our users online, to discuss their ideas in more detail, and to mentor other persons interested in adapting the innovations in their own settings. Several contributors also granted permission for tools that they developed to be reprinted in this volume. *Innovations in End-of-Life Care: Practical Strategies and International Perspectives* would not exist without their work and their willingness to share it.

Mildred Z. Solomon, EdD
Anna L. Romer, EdD
Karen S. Heller, PhD

Center for Applied Ethics and Professional Practice
Education Development Center, Inc.
Newton, Massachusetts

Part One

Introduction

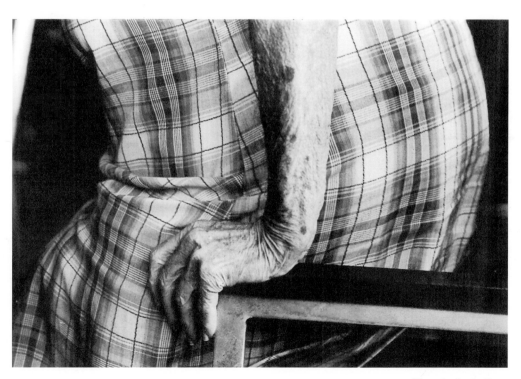

Photo by Jamie Cope

Introduction

Innovations in End-of-Life Care: Mission and Purpose

MILDRED Z. SOLOMON, EdD

*Education Development Center, Inc.,
Newton, Massachusetts*

In 1998, The Robert Wood Johnson Foundation, based in Princeton, New Jersey, funded the launch by Education Development Center, Inc. of a new online journal (www.edc.org/lastacts). Entitled Innovations in End-of-Life Care, *this multidisciplinary journal is a source of information for health care professionals who are interested in strengthening the capacity of the organizations in which they work to care better for dying patients and their families. In this chapter, Mildred Z. Solomon, EdD, editor-in-chief of* Innovations, *explains the rationale for the project and introduces this volume, a compilation of selected material published online over the last year.*

All over the world, people are developing better ways to provide care to the dying and to their families. Nearly 2500 health care professionals from more than 73 countries attended the most recent conference of the European Association for Palliative Care, held in September 1999 in Geneva, Switzerland.[1] The agenda was filled with presentations on research, and clinical and educational initiatives to ease patient suffering and support families. The Canadian Palliative Care Association has published a conceptual framework for establishing quality standards in palliative care,[2] and Canadian leaders are involved in a host of educational programs to support the development of palliative care services in Canada and abroad. In the United Kingdom, researchers are refining outcome measures and developing audit tools that are being tried out in hospitals and other kinds of health care settings throughout the United Kingdom and in many other countries.[3] The Italian government has allocated 450 billion lira, or roughly $238 million dollars, to enhance palliative-care and hospice services.[4] In Spain, as of 1998, an intensive investment of time and human resources has resulted in the establishment of 143 palliative-care services in many regions of the country.[5] Israel is hosting a conference on the intersection of end-of-life care and cultural diversity* and another on bereavement.†

---

*Palliative Care 2000: Palliative Care in Different Cultures. A Congress With the Collaboration of EAPC. Jerusalem, Israel. March 12–23, 2000.
†Sixth International Conference on Grief and Bereavement in Contemporary Society: Life, Grief, Coping and Continuity. Jerusalem, Israel. July 9–14, 2000.

In the United States, the Institute of Medicine, a charter organization of the National Academy of Sciences, Washington, D.C., and one of the nation's most important policy bodies for medicine and health, issued *Approaching Death: Improving Care at the End of Life*—a virtual call-to-arms to U.S. physicians and health care organizations.[6] More than 450 organizations have joined the Last Acts campaign, a national effort to improve the care of the dying, initiated by The Robert Wood Johnson Foundation. Many other philanthropic foundations also have committed themselves to supporting end-of-life initiatives.‡ Several medical specialty societies have developed principles to guide palliative-care improvement efforts,[7] and there are efforts focused on enhancing palliative-care knowledge and teaching skills of medical school faculty.§ A national task force offered recommendations to leaders of managed care organizations, calling on them to assess the impact of cost-containment measures on the quality of health care delivered to dying patients and to realign financial incentives to encourage more humane and competent palliative care.[8],‖

These examples only begin to scratch the surface of what is going on around the globe. Why all this attention? Numerous research studies have documented major inadequacies in the care that patients near the end of life and their families receive. It is now known, for example, that:

- Patients are dying in pain and suffering from a variety of other physical discomforts, despite the fact that medicines and therapeutics exist to control most symptoms near the end of life.[9-11] The problem is that medical and nursing education has been lacking and most health care organizations have not made pain and symptom management an institutional priority; in some parts of the world, access to the necessary drugs are limited by law or regulation.[12]
- In some countries, technologies are imposed upon patients that merely prolong the dying process, while simpler acts of care and support are not provided.[13,14]
- Depression, emotional suffering, and grief go unnoticed or unacknowledged.[15] This abandonment of the psychological aspects of death and dying affects health care providers' abilities to support patients and families; it also takes a toll on health care providers themselves, who frequently have no outlet or support for their own grief.
- In many places, there is poor continuity of care.[16,17] As patients move from tertiary care centers to nursing homes or hospices, they encounter new sets of health care professionals, who may not know their personal histories and who cannot shepherd families through the end-of-life period with confidence and ease.
- Hospice care, where it exists, is often underutilized.[18] Referral to a hospice of-

---

‡Grantmakers Concerned with Care at the End of Life, 400 West 59th Street, New York, NY 10019.
§The Harvard Medical School Program in Palliative Care Education. J. Andrew Billings, MD, and Susan D. Block, MD, program directors. Harvard Medical School, Boston, MA. Grant provided by The Robert Wood Johnson Foundation, Princeton, NJ, July 1998–June 2003.
‖For a copy, contact Stacy Piszcz by phone at: (617) 969-7100, extension 2388; by e-mail at: mcare@edc.org, or download with Adobe Acrobat Reader at: www.edc.org/CAE/meetingchallenge

ten occurs in the last few days of life, so that patients and families cannot receive the benefits that a hospice has to offer in terms of psychosocial support and help with life closure. Moreover, the hospice model and palliative care, in general, were developed originally to care for cancer patients; models for adapting hospice and palliative care for people suffering from other diseases are only in their infancy.[19]

Research in the 1990s documented the extent of the problems. If the extent of activity going on around the world is any indication, it is to be hoped the first decades of the 2000s will offer some remedies.

The reason for optimism is clear. In addition to the large amount of work being undertaken by palliative care specialists, specialty societies, and policymaking bodies, there are also many physicians, nurses, social workers, and pastoral counselors in hospitals, long-term care facilities, hospices, and home care agencies, who have become personally committed to the problems of end-of-life care and are actively engaged in being part of the solution. However, too often, these champions are working in isolation. Frequently, they are solitary advocates in systems that do not necessarily share their passion or that do not have the flexibility to change easily. These change agents run the risk of "burnout," and could benefit from exchange with like-minded professionals who share their passion for improving the care of the dying.

In 1998, The Robert Wood Johnson Foundation, funded the launch by the Education Development Center, Inc. of a new Web-based journal (www.edc.org/lastacts). Entitled *Innovations in End-of-Life Care*, this multidisciplinary journal seeks to be a source of information for health care professionals who are interested in strengthening the capacity of the organizations in which they work to care for dying patients and their families better.

The purpose of *Innovations* is to improve the quality of care provided to patients near the end of life and to their families, through the dissemination and critical examination of innovative practices being implemented throughout the world. By the term "innovations," the journal means to include practices that are new as well as those that have been ongoing for some time in one or more regions of the world, but that are not yet well known or adopted in other regions. The goal of such innovations should be to deliver more humane, more effective, more comprehensive, and/or more coordinated care, so that patients will experience enhanced comfort, higher physical functioning, and a greater sense of well-being. Innovations that aim to demedicalize the dying experience are particularly desired. For example, there is a special interest in innovations that help dying patients connect with their families and community, find spiritual meaning, or develop their own artistic expressions near the end of life.

There are already several palliative care journals in existence. *Innovations'* special niche is in focusing on the social and political processes, administrative actions, and organizational steps that were necessary for initiating and maintaining these improvements. The idea is to slow down or "unpack" the change process, so that other people can learn from and adapt these practices in their own settings. To give innovators the opportunity to describe the strategies they used, the barriers they encountered, and how they overcame those hurdles, we encourage contributors to offer what the ethnographer, Clifford Geertz, called, "thick description."[20] Sometimes we gather these thick descriptions through peer-reviewed authored papers and sometimes through an interview process, which results in a published dialogue between an *Innovations* editor and an innovator. Innovations featured in these interviews are always carefully selected and reviewed by the journal's associate editors and/or editorial board members prior to publication.

An important part of *Innovations'* mission is fostering cross-national and cross-cultural exchange. Every strategy that people invent to improve the care of the dying is based on explicit or implicit values about what would constitute good care near the end of life, as well as assumptions about the cause of the problem being addressed and how best to remedy it. Innovative practices are also shaped by how care is delivered and financed. Therefore, in every online issue, palliative care experts from around the world comment on the featured innovation, explaining how that intervention would, or would not, be relevant and/or adaptable in their countries, given their societal values and their systems of health care delivery and finance.

For example, in Volume 1, Number 1 about advance-care planning, reprinted here as Part Two, international commentators from Spain, Italy, Australia, the Netherlands and Israel, explain why advance directives are not widely used in their countries.[21-25] Their views stand in sharp contrast to predominant values expressed over the last 20 years in the United States. In the United States, from the first so-called "right-to-die" case in 1976 (the case of Karen Ann Quinlan)[26] right up to the 1995 publication of the results of the SUPPORT study[27] (the largest end-of-life care intervention in the United States to date), there has been a widespread assumption that enhancing patient self-determination, particularly through the use of advance directives, would be the best way to enhance end-of-life care. The juxtaposition of the prevailing US view with the international views in that same issue led to an editorial, which asked, "Why are advance directives a non-issue outside the United States?"[28] International and cross-cultural exchange is a helpful device for revealing the often unconscious assumptions that lead people to design one kind of innovation and not another.

Innovations' commitment to international and cross-cultural exchange is part of our explicit attempt to get at the values underlying innovation. Without that values discussion, we run the risk of becoming the technocrats that Daniel Callahan, one of the architects of American bioethics, recently warned against. With the recent surge in attention to the problem of end-of-life care and, as many specialty societies and other professional elites began inventing strategies for making improvements, Mr. Callahan opined, "Isn't that typically American? Why do we think that what we need is more innovation? The problem of end-of-life care is a problem of cultural values—how we think about death and dying, what relative weight we put on health, as opposed to other possible goods, how we think about our mortality and the suffering of others. It is not a technical problem in search of a technical fix."¶

¶Personal communication, Daniel Callahan, The Hastings Center, Garrison, NY.

Ultimately, the kind of exchange we have tried to promote online and in this volume is an exchange about how to bring more meaning to the inevitable, universal experience of death and dying. The innovations we seek to publish are not just changes in institutional policies and procedures, though often they are that. Each of them is selected because it holds promise for enhancing the comfort and dignity of dying persons and their families, or because it supports the dying and their loved ones as they struggle with spiritual and existential challenges.

The promising practice offered by Navah Harlow, MA, of Beth Israel Medical Center in New York City, which appears in Part Three of this volume, is a prime example.[29] Ms. Harlow invites families to write farewell letters to their loved ones. Although developed as a way of helping families articulate what treatment options they think their now-incapacitated loved ones would have wanted, the strategy has proved helpful in other ways as well. Writing these letters has helped families come to terms with dire prognoses, enabled the families to arrive at consensus about treatment options, and served as a way of saying goodbye to loved ones. The beautiful personal essay by Thomas Cassirer, in Part Five, is another example.[30] In "Separate and Yet Together: Living with a Spouse Suffering from Alzheimer's Disease," Professor Cassirer describes the ways in which he continuously reinvents his relationship with his wife, as she struggles with advancing dementia.

Daniel Callahan is right. The problem of death and dying is not a technical problem in need of a technical fix. Rather, it is a problem of values in search of personal insight, public self-examination, and institutional action. Champions working within health care organizations can do a lot to promote richer discourse and greater innovation. Indeed, physicians, nurses, social workers, and hospital clergy are the people best situated to ensure that patient and family needs get met.

This volume contains much for those champions to consider. It covers four themes we addressed during 1999: advance care planning, family-centered care, cancer pain management, and dementia. Contributors come from Australia, Germany, Israel, Italy, the Netherlands, Scotland, Spain, and the United States. Many contributors generously allowed us to reprint tools they developed to aid their innovations, and these appear in Appendix A. There are also selected bibliographies in Parts Two through Five for readers who want to pursue any of these topics in more depth. I am confident that readers will find these articles, interviews, tools, and resources highly motivating. It is hoped the ideas embedded within these materials will stimulate us to think about how, in our own ways and our own workplaces, we can each make a contribution to the care of the dying and their families.

REFERENCES

1. Time—100 days before the year 2000: VIth Congress of the European Association for Palliative Care, Geneva, Switzerland. September 22–24, 1999.
2. Ferris FD, Cummings I., eds. *Palliative Care: Towards a Consensus in Standardized Practice.* Ottawa, Ontario: Canadian Palliative Care Association, 1995.

3. Higginson IJ., ed. *Clinical Audit in Palliative Care.* Oxford, UK: Radcliffe Medical Press, 1993.
4. Toscani F, Romer AL. Using the STAS in a palliative care unit in Cremona, Italy. *J Palliative Med* 2000;3:237–242. [Originally published in *Innovations in End-of-Life Care* 2000;2(1): International Perspectives (www.edc.org/lastacts/)]
5. Centeno C, Heller K. Palliative care in Spain: An evolving model: *J Palliative Med* 2000;3:123–127. [Originally published in *Innovations in End-of-Life Care* 1999;1(5): International Perspectives (www.edc.org/lastacts)]
6. Institute of Medicine Committee on Care at the End of Life; Field MJ, Cassel CK, eds. *Approaching Death: Improving Care at the End of Life.* Washington, DC: National Academy Press, 1997.
7. Cassel CK, Foley KM. *Principles for Care of Patients at the End of Life: An Emerging Consensus Among the Specialties of Medicine.* New York: Millbank Memorial Fund, 1999.
8. Solomon MZ, Romer AL, Sellers D, Jennings B, and the National Task Force on End-of-Life Care in Managed Care. *Meeting the Challenge: Twelve Recommendations for Improving End-of-Life Care in Managed Care.* Newton, MA: Education Development Center, Inc., 1999.
9. The Study to Understand Prognoses and Preferences for Outcomes and Risks of Treatments (SUPPORT): A controlled trial to improve care for seriously ill hospitalized patients. *JAMA* 1995;274:1591–1597.
10. Ferrell BR, Dean GE, Grant M, Coluzzi P. An institutional commitment to pain management. *J Clin Oncol* 1995;13:2158–2165.
11. American Pain Society Task Force on Pain, Symptoms and End-of-Life Care [Mitchell M (Chair), Clery J, Ferrell B, Foley K, Payne R, Shapiro B.] Treatment of pain at the end of life: A position statement from the American Pain Society. *APS Bull* 1997;7(1):1,3.
12. Joranson DE. Guiding principles of international and federal laws pertaining to medical use and diversion of controlled substances. In: *Evaluation of the Import of Prescription Drug Diversion Control Systems on Medical Practice and Patient Care: Possible Implications for Future Research* [Monograph 131]. National Institute on Drug Abuse Technical Research, 1993:18–35.
13. Solomon MZ, O'Donnell L, Jennings B, Guilfoy V, Wolf S, Nolan K, Jackson R, Koch-Weser D, Donnelley S. Decisions near the end of life: Professional views on life-sustaining treatments. *Am J Pub Health* 1993;83:14–23.
14. Solomon MZ, Jennings B, Guilfoy V, Jackson R, O'Donnell L, Wolf SM, Nolan K, Koch-Weser D, Donnelley S. Toward an expanded vision of clinical ethics education: From the individual to the institution. *Kennedy Inst Ethics J* 1991;83(1):225–245.
15. Byock I. *Dying Well.* New York: Riverhead Books, 1997.
16. Institute of Medicine Committee on Care at the End of Life. Chapter 4. In: Field MJ, Cassel CK., eds. *Approaching Death: Improving Care at the End of Life.* Washington, DC: National Academy Press, 1997, pp. 107–115.
17. Steel K, Leff B, Vaitovas B. A home care annotated bibliography. *J Am Geriatric Soc* 1998;46:898–909.
18. National Hospice Organization, Committee on the Medicare Hospice Benefit and End-of-Life Care: Final Report to the Board of Directors. Arlington, VA: National Hospice Organization after Board of Directors.
19. National Hospice Organization. *Medical Guidelines for Determining Prognosis in Selected Non-Cancer Diseases,* 2nd ed. Arlington, VA: National Hospice Organization, 1996.

20. Geertz C. *Local Knowledge: Further Essays in Interpretive Anthropology.* New York: Basic Books, 1983.

21. Glick S. The truth, the whole truth, and nothing but the truth? In: Solomon MZ, Romer AL, Heller KS, eds. *Innovations in End-of-Life Care: Practical Strategies and International Perspectives.* Larchmont, NY: Mary Ann Liebert, Inc., 2000, pp. 39–42. [Originally published in *Innovations in End-of-Life Care* 1999;1(1): International Perspectives (www.edc.org/lastacts).]

22. Kristjanson L. Advance-care planning in the Australian context. In: Solomon MZ, Romer AL, Heller KS., eds. *Innovations in End-of-Life Care: Practical Strategies and International Perspectives.* Larchmont, NY: Mary Ann Liebert, Inc., 2000, pp. 43–46. [Originally published in *Innovations in End-of-Life Care* 1999;1(1): International Perspectives (www.edc.org/lastacts/).]

23. Nuñez Olarte JM. Cultural attitudes toward death and dying in Spain. In: Solomon MZ, Romer AL, Heller KS., eds. *Innovations in End-of-Life Care: Practical Strategies and International Perspectives.* Larchmont, NY: Mary Ann Liebert, Inc., 2000, pp. 47–51. [Originally published in *Innovations in End-of-Life Care* 1999;1(1): International Perspectives (www.edc.org/lastacts/).]

24. Ripamonte C. Speaking in a particular way. Individualizing communication for each patient. In: Solomon MZ, Romer AL, Heller KS., eds. *Innovations in End-of-Life Care: Practical Strategies and International Perspectives.* Larchmont, NY: Mary Ann Liebert, Inc., 2000, pp. 53–55. [Originally published in *Innovations in End-of-Life Care* 1999;1(1): International Perspectives (www.edc.org/lastacts/).]

25. Zylicz ZB. Limitations to advance directives. A Dutch view. In: Solomon MZ, Romer AL, Heller KS., eds. *Innovations in End-of-Life Care: Practical Strategies and International Perspectives.* Larchmont, NY: Mary Ann Liebert, Inc., 2000, pp. 57–61. [Originally published in *Innovations in End-of-Life Care* 1999;1(1): International Perspectives (www.edc.org/lastacts/).]

26. *In re* Quinlan. 1976. N.J. 10, 355. A.2d.647, cert. denied, 429 U.S. 922.

27. Solomon MZ. Why are advance directives a non-issue outside the United States? In Solomon MZ, Romer AL, Heller KS, eds. *Innovations in End-of-Life Care: Practical Strategies and International Perspectives.* Larchmont, NY: Mary Ann Liebert, Inc., 2000, pp. 13–18. [Originally published in *Innovations in End-of-Life Care* 1999;1(1): Editorial (www.edc.org/lastacts/).]

28. Harlow N. An interview with Navah Harlow, MA by AL Romer. In: Solomon MZ, Romer AL, Heller KS., eds. *Innovations in End-of-Life Care: Practical Strategies and International Perspectives.* Larchmont, NY: Mary Ann Liebert, Inc., 2000, pp. 69–71. [Originally published in *Innovations in End-of-Life Care* 1999;1(2): Featured Innovation (www.edc.org/lastacts/).]

29. Cassirer T. Separate and yet together: Living with a spouse suffering from Alzheimer's disease. In: Solomon MZ, Romer AL, Heller KS., eds. *Innovations in End-of-Life Care: Practical Strategies and International Perspectives.* Larchmont, NY: Mary Ann Liebert, Inc., 2000, pp. 145–150. [Originally published in *Innovations in End-of-Life Care* 1999;1(4): Personal Reflections (www.edc.org/lastacts/).]

Part Two

*Communication, Truth Telling, and
Advance Care Planning*

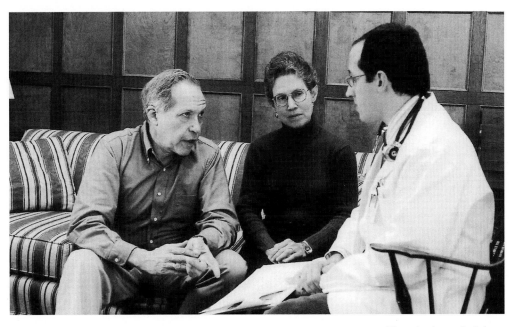

Photo by Aaron Sodickson

Why are Advance Directives a Non-Issue Outside the United States?

MILDRED Z. SOLOMON, EdD

Education Development Center, Inc.
Newton, Massachusetts

This section of *Innovations in End-of-Life Care: Practical Strategies and International Perspectives* does two things that, to our knowledge, have not been done together. First, we feature an American innovation that has succeeded in promoting the completion of advance directives among a startlingly high proportion of people in one geographic area. The Respecting Your Choices™ program, spearheaded by Bernard J. Hammes, PhD, in La Crosse, Wisconsin, has achieved what no other community in the United States, or elsewhere, can claim: Eighty-one percent of the people in that community have executed some form of advance directive and there is documentation of their wishes in the medical records.[1] Through a question-and-answer format in our Featured Innovation (see pages 19–38), we present an in-depth analysis of the processes and strategies that led to that outcome.

However, advance directives are not in use in most other countries, and this chapter sets out to explore why not. In the International Perspectives section (see pages 39–61), palliative care experts from Australia, Israel, Italy, the Netherlands, and Spain explain the ways in which health care decision making and end-of-life care are conceptualized and carried out in their countries. How is autonomy understood and to what extent is it emphasized? What do the clinicians, patients, and families in these countries see as the proper role of truth telling? What advice can we glean about how best to communicate with patients and families near the end of life?

Our goal is threefold: first, to let readers know of the most effective innovation, to date, that has succeeded in improving advance care planning in the United States; second, to shed light on the fundamental premises that have driven the emphasis on advance directives in the United States, with the hope that unpacking these assumptions can lead to the design of other, potentially complementary, strategies; and third, to inaugurate *Innovations in End-of-Life Care* as a place where contrasting perspectives are sought to ignite creative thinking and improve end-of-life care across very different cultures and health care delivery systems.

In the United States, the focus on advance directives can be traced directly back to the American emphasis on autonomy and truth telling. Advance directives were conceived as a way to ensure that patients' wishes would guide the kind of treatments they received near the end of life. These directives have come in two main forms: (1) highly specific documents, often called living wills or medical wills, that stipulate the sorts of treatments patients would or would not want, under various future medical circumstances; and (2) documents in which patients designate individuals to serve as their health care agents, or proxies, for some time in the future, when these patients are no longer able to speak for themselves.

Both living wills and the designation of health care agents have been highly promoted throughout the United States. Yet, our international guests find them, at best, moot. Reading across their commentaries, several points emerge.

SELF-DETERMINATION OR ACCESS TO SERVICES?

In the United States, historically, the problem of end-of-life care has been framed as one of self-determination. In many other countries, the problem has been framed as one of providing services.

Beginning with the 1976 case of Karen Ann Quinlan, a young woman in a persistent vegetative state whose parents wanted her ventilator discontinued, end-of-life care in the United States has essentially been conceived as a process of ethical analysis and personal decision making. Until very recently, policy makers and bioethicists had framed the challenge of improving end-of-life care as one of getting better at ascertaining with as much precision as possible exactly what patients themselves would want. More recently, in the United States, and particularly with the publication of the Institute of Medicine report, *Approaching Death*,[2] the focus on advance directives has shifted to the broader, less document-driven concept of advance care planning. There is also growing attention to the development of standards of care, care delivery, and clinician preparation.[3-7] Nevertheless, the strong historical emphasis in the United States on self-determination has focused tremendous attention on making choices about what particular treatment modality someone does or does not want. This focus, in turn, has led down a highly legalistic path.

In other countries, the challenge has been framed not as one of choice and self-determination, but as how best to provide a comprehensive set of services and how to prepare physicians, nurses, and others with the skills necessary for delivering those services. I do not mean to overromanticize the state of palliative care services outside the United States, nor to gloss over important variations in the quality of that care both within countries and between countries. However, it is helpful to acknowledge that, fundamentally, there have been very different conceptual frameworks for approaching what is, essentially, a common global problem.

THE IMPORTANCE OF RELATIONSHIPS

Our commentators live in countries with national public health systems, a strong emphasis on primary care, and less geographic mobility among their patient populations. A great deal of care is provided at home by general practitioner–nurse teams. As a consequence, patients are better known by their physicians and more trusting of the doctor–patient relationship. In this context, dying becomes a natural part of the continuum of care. Thus, strengths and weaknesses in communication and advance care planning are, to a very great extent, functions of how a health care system is organized. As Zbigniew Zylicz, MD, PhD, of the Netherlands puts it, "You cannot see communication separately from the system."

Long-term relationships between general practitioners, patients, and families, coupled with the existence of palliative care services, solve many of the communication problems that, in the United States, advance care directives are intended to ameliorate. As Linda Kristjanson, PhD, of Australia explains, once the decision to accept palliative care is made, "people accept that certain things won't happen," the "resuscitation matter dissolves," and patient, family, and health care team address each end-of-life question, such as tube feedings or the use of antibiotics, as these issues arise. In this context, she continues, "You know your patients, the relationship is very individualized, thus an advance directive would be seen as a legalistic document that would be incongruent in the context of the relationship."

FOR LACK OF A CRYSTAL BALL

Furthermore, advance directives, particularly living wills, which can suffer from too much specificity, assume that patients' wishes will be stable over time, as their health changes. As Dr. Zylicz points out, "Patients create and sign living wills, when they are healthy. For us, it is important to find out what the patient wants at the moment when he or she is very ill." Dr. Zylicz' concerns are borne out empirically, because there is research suggesting that, as people become more debilitated, they are willing to accept more limitations in their quality of life.

Is it possible to know what one would want in some future time, in a wholly different situation? As Juan Núñez Olarte, MD, PhD, of Spain puts it, "We change marriages, we change political sides, we change religious convictions. And we expect, when we are facing death, we are not going to change?"

Furthermore, many physicians point out that what was said in a specific treatment directive should not automatically be assumed to apply to that patient's current situation. Shimon Glick, MD, of Israel tells the story of a young Bedouin patient who had completely reversible pneumonia but, because he had an advance directive asking not to be intubated, he was allowed to die. Dr. Glick asks us to consider, "Is this really what the patient would have wanted?"

CONCEPTS OF AUTONOMY AND TRUTH TELLING
VARY ACROSS CULTURES

The apparent lack of truth telling in such countries as Italy and Spain, where patients are not routinely told their cancer diagnoses or prognoses of impending death, has been highly criticized. Yet, commentaries by Carla Ripamonti, MD, and Drs. Núñez Olarte and Glick shed light on the nature of truth-telling in their countries, and the story is more complex. For example, research that Dr. Núñez Olarte and his colleagues have done on patients' attitudes demonstrates that a very significant number of patients either do not want to know their prognoses, or are ambivalent about such prognoses. The art of providing palliative care depends, in part, on understanding just how much information each patient wants and modulating one's response to fit with that patient's needs and expectations. As Dr. Ripamonti of Italy says, "We have some patients who want to know their situation exactly and explicitly, so we speak exactly with them. And we give all our patients the opportunity to ask everything. We try to understand what, and how much, they want to know."

Our commentators' findings are similar to the findings that researchers have discovered among different cultural groups within the United States. Blackhall, et al.[8] as well as Koenig,[9] Koenig and Gates-William,[10] and others[11,12] have found that many dying patients do not want to know the details of their prognosis, nor want to make their own autonomously derived decisions about their treatment options. For many such patients, family needs, obligations and responsibilities are of greater importance.

Such cross-cultural insights are helpful for articulating a more nuanced concept of autonomy. Dr. Glick says, "While I think one should tell the truth to patients in general, there are times when I don't, and I think there are times when patients don't want it, and they're very upset when you do."

"Autonomy," Dr. Núñez Olarte concludes, "does not mean assaulting patients with truth, or assaulting them with informed consent, or assaulting them with advance directives." These sentiments echo advice that Dr. Benjamin Freedman, the late Canadian researcher, provided when he suggested that health care providers "offer" truth, but not impose it.[13]

KINDNESS

Autonomy is not a command, but rather an invitation, a freeing of space for the possibility of self-fulfilling action. When autonomy is wielded like a club, it can be cruel and destructive. In contrast, Dr. Ripamonti talks about speaking in a *particular* way—a way that helps a patient arrive at his or her own sense of the prognosis. Furthermore, Dr. Ripamonti expects and accepts what others might merely dismiss, with frustration and exasperation, as "denial." "You could have a patient," she explains, "who clearly knows her prognosis but, when she feels better, she believes that death is not near. One day we are able to accept death; the day after, we are not."

> *Autonomy is not a command, but rather an invitation, a freeing of space for the possibility of self-fulfilling action.*

What all these commentators share is a commitment to individualizing decisions—not through prior advance directives about a hypothetical time, but in the moment—a moment that is inevitably conflicted, uncertain, and fraught with ambivalence, one that requires acts of human kindness more than treatment directives.

In fact, if we look closely at what Respecting Your Choices™ accomplished in La Crosse, Wisconsin, it was exactly that—better ways to ensure that conversations took place within families and among patients, families, and health care providers. Dr. Hammes emphasizes that the goal is not to get people to fill out paperwork, but to use that task as an impetus to ensure that conversations take place. Most of the components in the Respecting Your Choices™ program involved helping family members talk amongst themselves and with their health care professionals. In the US health care system, we may need to work harder to ensure that this happens, because, unfortunately, we can not assume long-standing relationships with our physicians or continuity of care as patients move across care settings. Dr. Hammes' group has demonstrated one very effective strategy for enhancing communication in a context where it is harder to win. I invite you to read about what he has achieved and to consider how it might be adapted for your community.

REFERENCES

1. Hammes BJ, Rooney BL. Death and end-of-life planning in one midwestern community. *Arch Int Med* 1998;158:383–390.
2. Institute of Medicine Committee on Care at the End of Life. In: *Approaching Death: Improving Care at the End of Life.* Field MJ, Cassel CK, eds. Washington, DC: National Academy Press, 1997.
3. Last Acts Precepts of Palliative Care. Developed by the Task Force on Palliative Care, as part of the Last Acts: Care and Caring at the End of Life Campaign. Web site: http://www.lastacts.org, 1997.
4. American Geriatric Society. Measuring quality of care at the end of life: A statement of principles. *J Am Geriatric Soc* 1997;45:526–527.
5. American Pain Society Task Force on Pain, Symptoms and End-of-Life Care. Max M, chair, Clery J, Ferrell B, Foley K, Payne R, Shapiro, B. Treatment of pain at the end of life: A position statement from the American Pain Society. *APS Bull* 1997;7(1).
6. American Board of Internal Medicine. Educational Resource Document: *Caring for the Dying: Identification and Promotion of Physician Competency.* ABIM Web site: http://www.abim.org, 1996.
7. American Association of Colleges of Nursing. Peaceful death: Recommended competencies and curricular guidelines for end-of-life nursing care. In: *Educational Standards and Special Projects.* AACN Web site: http://www.aacn.nche.edu/deathfin.htm.
8. Blackhall L, Murphy, S, Frank, G, Michel V, Azen, S. Ethnicity and attitudes toward patient autonomy. *JAMA* 1995;274 (10):820–825.
9. Koenig B. Cultural diversity in decision making about care at the end of life. In: *Approaching Death: Improving Care at the End of Life.* Field MK, Cassel CK, eds. Washington, DC: National Academy Press, 1997, pp. 363–382.
10. Koenig B, Gates-Williams J. Understanding cultural difference in caring for dying patients. *Western J Med* 1995;163(3):244–249.

11. Ersk M, Kagawa-Singer M, Barnes D, Blackhall L, Koenig BA. Multicultural considerations in the use of advance directives. *Oncol Nurs Forum* 1998;25(10): 1683–1690.
12. Cultural issues in palliative care. Section 10 in: *Oxford Textbook of Palliative Medicine*. Doyle D, Hanks GWC, MacDonald N, eds. Oxford, UK: Oxford University Press, 1998, pp. 777–801.
13. Freedman B. Offering truth: One ethical approach to the uninformed cancer patient. *Arch Int Med* 1993;153(5):572–576.

The Lessons from
Respecting Your Choices™

An Interview with BERNARD J. HAMMES, PhD

Gunderson Lutheran Medical Center
La Crosse, Wisconsin

Bernard J. Hammes, PhD, director of medical humanities at Gundersen Lutheran Medical Center and his colleagues on the La Crosse Area Medical Center's Task Force on Advance Directives, Wisconsin, wanted to make sure that patient and family values and preferences would guide end-of-life treatment decisions in La Crosse, Wisconsin. The result of their efforts is Respecting Your Choices™: An Advance Directive Education Program, a community-wide advance directive education project. An evaluation of this multidimensional intervention revealed that a full 81 percent of decedents in the community had documentation in the medical records indicating their treatment preferences and values or their choice of health care agents who could speak for them when they were no longer able to speak for themselves.[1] This finding stands in stark contrast to all other efforts in the United States to promote advance directives. Nationwide, only between 15 to 25 percent of outpatients in the United States have reported completing advance directives and even fewer patients actually have their documents in the medical records.[2]

What is equally impressive is that chart review and retrospective interviews with family members demonstrated that nearly all the deceased patients received treatments that were consistent with their expressed wishes.[1] Other American studies have documented extremely poor concordance between patient' preferences and the treatments that their physicians[3] and their spouses thought they wanted.[4]

The contrast between the La Crosse experience and other efforts to promote advance directives in the United States is so sharp that we invited Dr. Hammes to discuss with us how he and his colleagues instigated such a comprehensive cultural change in the practice of medicine in their community. One feature that stands out here is that four local health care systems that compete in other domains chose to work together in the service of this educational venture and, as a result, developed a program that has its own community identity. The four health systems with staffs that worked together to spawn this effort were the Franciscan Health System, the Gundersen Clinic, Ltd., the Lutheran Health System-Lacrosse, and the Skemp Clinic, Ltd. These organizations have now consolidated into Franciscan Skemp Healthcare and Gundersen Lutheran.

The interview with Dr. Hammes which follows was conducted by Anna L. Romer, EdD.

RESPECTING YOUR CHOICES™ AND ITS GOALS

Anna L. Romer: *What is the innovation you developed?*

Bernard Hammes: Respecting Your Choices™ is a comprehensive advance directive education program formulated by the La Crosse Area Medical Centers' Task Force on Advance Directives, of which I'm a member. The components are:

- locally developed patient-education materials
- availability of these materials throughout the community
- training agendas and resources for educating a large core group of nonphysician educators
- access to advance directive educators at all health care organizations in the community
- common policies and practices of maintaining and using advance directive documents, including broad physician involvement
- documentation of advance directives in each patient's medical record and systems in place to ensure that this information "travels" with the patient across care settings.

ALR: *What were your goals in designing this innovation? What did you hope to achieve?*

BH: From the very beginning, there were a few things we felt were very important. One was not just to focus on the technical completion of documents, but rather to engage patients and their families as units. Our approach was to engage the patient, along with those who are close to the patient. It could be friends, it could be a religious group. It could be anyone. The question we asked was, "Who would be those people the patient would want at the bedside making decisions and supporting the patient?" We felt that should really be the locus of education.

The goal of education would be, first of all, to help these people understand what options and decisions might be faced, help them reflect on those decisions, work through those issues, and then both make decisions and communicate these decisions to each other and ultimately to the health professionals. How that was communicated was probably best in writing, but we left it open to some variation. The most important thing was that whatever was written down clearly reflected and communicated the patient's preferences.

Now there are obvious advantages of completing a legal document, particularly a power of attorney, for health care. But even that might vary from place to place, depending on what state statutes require and other kinds of rules and regulations of the law.

ALR: *Did you have other goals?*

BH: In addition to these primary goals, we wanted to assure patients and families that our systems would be able to track and make use of these documents and preferences. We wanted to be able to promise that any documents that they generated, through our assistance or on their own, would be put into the medical record reliably and would be retrievable and available, and then, finally, that those documents would be carefully considered in any decision making. We needed to have health professionals who understood how to implement those preferences and decisions.

From the very beginning of Respecting Your Choices™, we didn't want to do just a lot of exposure and education. We wanted to make sure that we could follow through on the implicit promise one makes when one solicits patient and family input. We wanted to be able to stand behind that promise, basically saying, "we want you to think about this, and we'll help you think about this, and if you do think about it, and tell us what your preferences are, we will look at that, and we will take it into account when making decisions."

PILOT PROGRAM THAT LED TO RESPECTING YOUR CHOICES™

ALR: *What steps did you take to initiate this innovation at your institution?*

BH: The project was informed by a pilot program that we ran in La Crosse between 1986 and 1991 called, If I Only Knew. The pilot program was an effort to develop a curriculum and education for chronic dialysis patients. We hoped to elicit from them their ideas about when they would want treatment withheld or, under what circumstances they would want treatment withheld, particularly focusing on cardiopulmonary resuscitation (CPR) and of course, dialysis.

So we asked the typical things: What kind of material would we have to use? Who would do the education? When would it be done? How would it be done? The pilot really helped us understand how to integrate that kind of advance care planning program into patient care.

ALR: *How did you finance the pilot?*

BH: We got a small grant from one of the local hospital foundations, and we got permission from both the dialysis unit and the hospital to use staff time to do this. Basically, we asked, "We educate patients on nutrition, we educate them about all other kinds of things, don't we need to educate them about these kinds of decisions? Because many of these patients are going to face them. Why is this different than any other kind of education we do for patients?" We convinced administrators that this kind of education was a responsible thing to do and something that we should offer patients. So we got permission to use staff and we got some extra money from the hospital foundation to pay for some of the materials.

ALR: *How many patients were you working with in the pilot?*

BH: At that time, I believe, we had a constant population of about 60 to 80 hemodialysis patients. It's a nice population to work with, because these patients are, in one sense, outpatients. And yet, they're on life support, and they are interacting with health professionals frequently and over lengthy periods of time. So the kind of relationship and opportunity are there to do these kinds of things, which gets a little bit trickier with other groups of patients, simply because the exposure and interaction may not be as frequent.

ALR: *Was there an evaluation component of that pilot?*

BH: The simple evaluation was just to do a pre- and post-test of the number of advance directives that we did. Prior to the program, only two percent of our dialysis patients had written advance directives. After two years, 46 percent of our dialysis patients had advance directives. We looked in their records and counted what they had. Physicians reported that they had a much easier time making these decisions with the patients or families than they had before the program.

    We found that, particularly with the dialysis patients, even with patients whose written advance directives do not become necessary to use because they remain competent, these previous discussions about values and preferences put patients and families in a better position to consider those issues when they faced decisions to withhold or stop treatment as competent patients.

ALR: *Can you give us an example?*

BH: Actually, it touched my family because my stepfather was one of the dialysis patients involved in the pilot. As a competent patient, he made a decision to stop dialysis. I was a little bit surprised, because this was a man who typically deferred decisions to my mother and, prior to that, to his former wife. He was a rather passive man, in decision making anyway. So when he, himself, made this decision quite quickly, I was very surprised and later asked my mom if she could give me any insight into this decision. She referred back to some of the things that had happened in the dialysis unit, discussing issues like CPR and other patients stopping treatment. These things helped him reflect on what he would or would not want in the future. I can only conjecture, because I was never able to ask him, that because of those experiences he had previously thought through what he would or would not want. Then when he was actually confronted with that decision, he was able to reach a conclusion and make a decision very quickly.

ALR: *How did the pilot inform your process, in designing Respecting Your Choices™, the community-wide intervention?*

BH: One reason we were able to make that big step is that our pilot served as evidence that this could be done, and how it could be done. We used that as a basis to explain to physicians and other health professionals what we did in a small population of people and how it worked.

It was particularly helpful, since one of the nephrologists was the president of one of the largest organizations, and he was willing to say to his physician colleagues, "It's a lot better to talk with patients and their families who have thought about these issues in advance; we have a lot less conflict and people feel more confident about their decisions." We also had data from the dialysis program to share with physicians. Data are always helpful when talking with medical groups—to say, "Here's what we did, how we did it, and the outcome." So, that kind of success on a small scale really helped convince skeptics or people who weren't so sure that there was value in doing this.

There's another thing that I didn't really understand until it happened. Our educational goals—understanding, reflection, communication and discussion, rather than the advance directive document itself—were very positively received by physicians. That wasn't anything we planned—it wasn't a strategy—but when I started to talk about the program I realized two things very quickly. First, we have physicians who say "documents don't help me," but who supported the concept of the program. When you can mostly deliver on that—patients and families are better prepared because of the process they've been through—physicians can support that. Even physicians who still oppose advance directives have a hard time publicly objecting to our goals since they are such an accepted part of informed consent.

THE IMPORTANCE OF TRAINING

ALR: *Were there other features that were important to your success?*

BH: One thing we learned in the pilot and carried through was the importance of having trained staff to do these conversations. We developed a day-and-a-half training in-service and only nonphysicians who have done the in-service are allowed to do advance directive education. We developed an educator manual, the *Respecting Your Choices™ Training Manual*, with 12 chapters that we use in those trainings and that can serve as resources for our counselors later.[5]

ALR: *Who gets trained at these in-services?*

BH: I would say the largest group of people is social workers, who work in hospitals, nursing homes, hospices, home health care, county health departments, and a few in ambulatory care. Then, it probably gets evenly divided between the next two groups—chaplains and nurses. The fourth group is a variety of people from the general community, who serve as volunteers for hospitals or other kinds of organizations.

ALR: *Do they all get the same training?*

BH: They all get the same training. Generally, the volunteers are people who are college educated, who have other kinds of professional training and experience, in terms of communication and human relations.

ALR: *What happens in the training?*

BH: The first morning, we lay out the general concepts and go into the psychology of end-of-life planning, language issues, and what kinds of medical issues are most important to talk about. We attempt to broaden the idea of what should be in this conversation and really focus on this as a process with goals of understanding, reflection, and communication and discussion. One key piece is that we recommend that the counselors go home and talk about their values and preferences for end-of-life care with their family members as part of the training, because we believe that grappling with these tough issues oneself is a prerequisite for facilitating that discussion with others. In the afternoon, the educators focus on their own knowledge, values, and beliefs in small and large group discussions. The goal is to reflect on what they heard in the morning, to integrate personal and professional beliefs, and to resolve and clarify their questions.

One week elapses between the first and second days of training and, during that time, educators complete a take-home exam, read the training manual, and complete a "power of attorney for health care" document for themselves or for a fictitious character. During the second half-day of training, the take-home exam is corrected, and the "power of attorney for health care" document is reviewed, but most of the morning is spent in role playing advance care planning discussions. The training ends with a final exam, which requires educators to outline how they would deal with three cases.

ALR: *How many people are you training each year now?*

BH: We train approximately 50 to 60 people a year. To date, we've trained more than 300 people as advance directive educators. Now, we're talking about just our local geographic area. I liken it to a CPR training or advanced cardiac life-support training. We do at least one additional in-service or update every year for people who have already been trained because there are new things—changes, and new ideas. So, we keep a list of names and addresses of people who have been trained, and we stay in contact with them through letters and other correspondence, such as sending articles that may be helpful to these people. Most recently, we developed a new "power of attorney for health care" form, and we did a two-hour in-service on that, in which the participants were allowed to comment, as educators, on the proposed draft, and we made additional changes.

SUSTAINING THE PROGRAM

ALR: *It sounds as though you had extensive physician support and input from early on that was key to getting the program going. What else is necessary to build and sustain this kind of program over time?*

BH: I think one of the things people need to understand (and that I feel painfully, sometimes every day) is that this is a program that needs to be managed. It's a very large system, and it requires constant attention and improvement. We have done a number of quality improvement projects, which really has been very important in making sure that a good program, in fact, works. This is something I probably can't emphasize too much. My experience has taught me that no matter how well designed a program is, implementing it is never smooth or perfect.

> *I think one of the things people need to understand (and that I feel painfully, sometimes every day) is that this is a program that needs to be managed. It's a very large system, and it requires constant attention and improvement. My experience has taught me that no matter how well designed a program is, implementing it is never smooth or perfect.*

ALR: *What quality indicators do you employ to assess the impact of your program?*

BH: Five years ago we sat down and looked at how advance directive education worked at our hospital. We identified two big areas in which we felt the system was not working properly. Then we developed two tools to measure our impact on them.

The Decision Tree Script

One area was the conversation that was occurring between the nurse and the patient when a patient got into a particular unit in the hospital. We felt that there were problems there, so we did some surveying of nurses regarding their practice and knowledge. We found a wide variation of practice and knowledge among nurses in talking with patients about advance directive documents and their treatment preferences. Although some nurses were very good, others were clearly inadequately prepared to conduct this kind of communication, despite prior training.

So, that was something we felt we needed to correct, and we had to come up with a strategy. Rather than going through another round of in-services and education for the hospital nursing staff, we developed a script with a decision tree for nurses to use.

Then we went back after nine months of implementing this script and decision tree and used the same tool to measure practice and knowledge, and what we found was a fairly consistent pattern of knowledge and practice.

The "Green Sleeve"

The other example is much simpler. We put the advance directive document and our education record in a "green sleeve" and, when a patient is hospitalized, those materials are supposed to be brought into the unit record. (This is literally a translucent, green plastic envelope that holds 8 × 11" sheets of paper.)

So, if you can imagine your hospital chart being in a folder, down in a file room, and, if you were brought into the hospital, that folder would be brought up to where your bed was in the nursing unit, and, if you had an advance directive, it would be in the "green sleeve." That green sleeve is now supposed to go in the ring binder that is your active chart while you're in the hospital.

The green sleeve moves to you, so to speak, from the file folder; it now becomes part of your immediate hospital record so that it's available and obvious to the health professionals caring for you during that hospitalization.

Well, that was the procedure outlined in our policy, and one question that came up was: "Do we do that all the time?" What we found is that, again, there was a lot of variation in practice. This time, it was based on individual misunderstandings, so, in a particular unit, one unit secretary might be very good at it and another secretary in the same unit may not do it at all. So the system only worked part of the time. We found that the policy was written in such a way that it led to misunderstanding. It was a simple matter of rewriting the policy in less ambiguous terms and then doing a little more education. We then went back and measured compliance and had nearly 100 percent compliance.

POTENTIAL BARRIERS

ALR: *Were there other barriers to implementing this advance care planning program?*

BH: Well, one of the things that very much concerned people was how this would be perceived by the community. One potential concern was that there would be a perception that we were doing this program for economic reasons, since it was being developed and promoted by health organizations.

Our answer, ultimately, was, "Look, if patients don't want care, and they tell us they don't want care, that's the primary motivation here. If that saves money, that saves money. If it doesn't save money, it doesn't save money." That consequence, the economic consequence, is irrelevant to what is the right thing to do. Again, I think emphasizing the respect of the individual's values really became a very strong message, which people saw as the overwhelming guiding ethical principle of the program. So, that broke down those kinds of community concerns and barriers.

The other concern was that religious communities might oppose this kind of program on theological, moral grounds, and think that what we were after was something akin to killing people.

ALR: *How did you address that?*

BH: We had a member of the clergy serve on our task force, and she became a liaison to the religious community. We have two bishops in our city, one a Roman Catholic and the other a Lutheran bishop. We approached both of them and talked with them about what we were trying to do, and asked them to give support for the program. In fact, we asked them to encourage clergy in their denominations to come to the training we were providing so that this kind of education could be conducted and carried out in churches throughout our area.

They responded positively and issued a joint letter to their clergy indicating their support for this program, in helping patients and their families think about end-of-life issues, and they encouraged their clergy to think about participating in this training.

ALR: *Were there already relationships in place here? This sounds too smooth to be true.*

BH: [Laughs] Well, yes, there were. One of the four major health care facilities that worked with us on this program is a Catholic facility. So, that was clearly an important factor in the support, and the hospitals and health institutions in this community are in fact, the biggest employers. They are major institutions in this city and, because of that, they have close and frequent contact with other institutions, including the churches. So, I don't want to say that this happened in a matter of a few minutes. This took months to negotiate and consider and think through, but I think it's part of the way the program was constructed, which is, we were really focused on trying to elicit from individuals their desires and their values.

ALR: *So it sounds as though you came to them early enough in the process.*

BH: We certainly had a very good idea of what we were going to do. The theme that we kept hammering at was that this really was an effort on the part of the hospitals to respect the values that individuals and families hold.

When we ran into certain people who held strong views on withdrawal of treatment, they felt, for example, that nutrition should never be withheld—our response was, "We're not trying to promote any particular value or view here about this, except the value of respecting the individual's choice. So if people feel very strongly about certain kinds of decisions, we want to know that, and we want clinicians to be able to respect those values."

I think we were able to deflect any major criticism of the health organizations or the program by focusing on our objective—to respect individuals' choices.

Our major concern as health professionals is to know when individuals do want us to do that and when they don't want us to do that, particularly if they can't tell us. We don't want to make that kind of mistake for an individual. So, we deflect it and say, "Look, if you have objections and think that withholding of nutrition and hydration should be made illegal, then you need to take that up with the state legislators or you need to take that up with the courts. It's not something we can solve; we can only do as much as we can to make sure that we make a good decision for each individual patient we care for."

ALR: *How do you respond to past research that showed that advance directives don't influence practice or family members' or clinicians' understandings of what patients would have wanted?*

BH: One of the issues that often comes up about advance directives is, "Well, you know, patients write these things down, but that's not what families actually do, and then physicians always follow the family." And I think that experience is actually pretty accurate.

So then the question is, "Why should I write these things down in a document when my family may not even follow these things, or the physician may not follow these things because the family doesn't support them or is anguishing over them, anyway?" I think that is a huge question, so at least part of our experience is that, in one sense, the intellectual clarification of values doesn't necessarily lead to the kind of decision making that might be implied.

So, I think there's a central issue here of how do you get people to act on their values, as opposed to just recognizing them? It has struck us, at least in La Crosse, that when families are anguishing about what is the right thing to do, that in their gut, what each individual is really saying is, "How can I be a good person, a loving son or daughter or whatever in making this kind of decision?" And that question hasn't been answered in the process of advance care planning.

FOCUS ON RELATIONSHIPS, NOT ABSTRACT VALUES

ALR: *How do you get people to focus on that question?*

BH: We reframe the conversation a bit and make it a more personal conversation. We say, "You know, if something were to happen to you, [if] you had a massive brain injury, what would you want your son or daughter to do for you? What would it mean for them to be good care providers and loving sons and daughters, if you could never recover from that brain injury?" In this way, the focus is really on relationships and not on abstract values.

ALR: *How do people respond to that kind of approach?*

BH: You need to have someone who can create an emotionally safe environment which allows a group of people who love each other to discuss these questions. This is why I think the training of people to have these conversations is so important. We call the people we train counselors or educators, but in a sense, they're guides and facilitators. This trained person has to make the family or patient comfortable and feel safe and then help them frame the questions in a way which are, in this sense, very personal.

ALR: *Your thinking is so different from the usual language and sets of assumptions that I think underlie many conversations about advance directives.*

BH: Right. One of the things that we notice, and again, this is more anecdotal in a sense, but one of the contrasts that we found in our advance directive study,[1] was that about 15 percent of the documents were done with attorneys. And there's this curious phenomenon that, often, those documents lead us to indecision. It's not because the documents are done improperly. It's because the documents are done by attorneys who haven't had this kind of a discussion with patients and families.

Just recently, I was asked to come and talk with a family that had a "power of attorney for health care," which even had some fairly good instructions in it. It was done eight years ago, so there's been plenty of time for family discussion, but when I asked the family what kind of conversation they had had about these issues with the author, who was now a patient, they said, "Well, we never talked about this." Some of them, even though they were named in the document, weren't really familiar with the document at all. So here we have this legal document, which provides minimal assistance in making decisions because this conversation had never occurred.

ALR: *So this brings us back to your first-stated goal of promoting understanding, reflection, and communication about values and preferences, rather than completing a document.*

INTERNATIONAL APPLICABILITY

ALR: *How would what you've done be useful in countries where there are no laws legalizing advance directives and where there isn't such an emphasis on individual autonomy, but families might have need for some guidance around these communication issues? Can you speak to that?*

BH: Well, first of all, I'm not sure that advance care planning is necessary everywhere. We have minority cultural groups in our own community on which, after a lot of thought, we decided we would not really focus any education. In particular, we have a group of H'mong from Southeast Asia and we have another relatively distinct group of Amish. These are two fairly sizable, identifiable cultural groups in our immediate geographic area. We had some conversations about what our obligations were to provide education about advance care planning to these groups. Our ultimate conclusion was that it would almost be disrespectful.

ALR: *Why?*

BH: Because advance care planning, at least as we approach it in this country, is really predicated on individual autonomy. And these cultures don't seem to hold that as a central value. I'm not saying they don't have it at all, it's just that it's not a central value for them the way it is for the more predominant culture in the United States. So, to go in and say, "You know, we want to respect your choices as individuals," is a little bit disrespectful of the fact that people within each of these groups may make decisions in a different way. Their way may be very hierarchical, and very patriarchal, and you know, each of us may have views on whether that's a good or a bad thing, but people within that system value it, accept it, and work within it.

The other part of it is that they have fairly well-established views about death and dying that guide them, from a value point of view, in knowing when to continue and when to stop medical care. So, unlike many of us in the dominant American culture who ask, "Gee, what are our values about this?" they *know* what their values are as a group.

ALR: *Have you run into problems of decision making with members of these groups?*

BH: No. We have not seen members of either of these cultures struggle greatly with these issues as family members approach death. To impose another system on them, and say, "You should change your system and now adapt ours" would be disrespectful. I reviewed some educational material done by a group, which had developed a videotape on advance care planning and advance directives, and the group did the video in English, Spanish, and H'mong. My comment was that you're taking a very specific, predominantly American, United States, culturally bound concept, and you're developing a scripted educational program to be provided through a video format, and you're simply translating the words and the concepts into H'mong, but that's not going to be intelligible. They'll understand the words, but the concepts and the values that you're promoting here are foreign. So, I had objections to that approach.

Now, making end-of-life decisions is still always hard because it's inherently filled with grief and sadness and complexity about what the choices are. I mean, those things are hard and there's nothing anyone can do about that.

ADVANCE CARE PLANNING

What advance care planning does is to lay out a set of relationships, values, and processes for knowing how to approach these decisions for individual people who live in a culture like ours, in which these things are not well understood or where there may be a lot of differences in opinion. That doesn't necessarily mean that every culture has those problems, and where this isn't an issue, advance care planning may be less germane.

The other comment I would have is that, nevertheless, we have to be sensitive to the fact that, even within cultures where end-of-life decision making is well-established, there can be variation or change. So, for example, we have many H'mong now who have become quite Westernized, and, in some sense, have given up many of their traditional values and relationships. Here, then, for someone who may have H'mong ancestry and family ties, it may become quite appropriate to do advance care planning.

ALR: *Thus far, you have been describing advance care planning as setting up a process and making values more transparent for people who live in a heterogeneous culture where things are less clear and where these values haven't been explicit. This brings up the issue of people wondering, "How will I know when my relative is actually dying?" Do you think of that as part of advance care planning, helping people anticipate and know? Or, is that just being a good doctor?*

BH: Well, in one sense, if you think about our current dilemma with technological care, fitting into the category of someone who is dying is, in some cases, a choice. So it is part of the advance care discussion.

For example, if I told my family, "If I reach a point where I'm largely unconscious and unresponsive, and I will never recover," when I tell them not to treat me, what I'm really saying is, "I want you to treat me as a dying person at that point," when, in fact, it may be technically possible to sustain biological life for long periods of time. So, my values about what is and is not important help define, in that particular instance, whether my family in a loving relationship, should treat me as a dying person or a person who has some life yet to live. So, I'm setting up a perspective of reality that is really driven by values and not by, say, some science.

It's really an interesting philosophical question. This is where my background does come into play. There are different cultural definitions and understandings of when people are dead. In some cultures, death doesn't occur for many, many days after the heart stops, because they believe that the soul inhabits the body and stays there for periods of time. So, one of the things that we need to understand and sometimes we forget, is that our science doesn't give us answers to these questions. They are not arbitrary, but they are ultimately realities that we create through a host of information and perspectives, and some of those perspectives are values. And by that, I'm separating them from something you scientifically go out and determine. They are driven by values and personal experiences, and not by objective, scientific measure.

TRUTH TELLING

ALR: *You mentioned earlier that you thought discussing advance-care planning might be disrespectful in some cultural contexts. How does this notion connect with a concern about informing patients that they are dying?*

BH: My perspective is that there may be and can be tremendous variation within cultures. In cultures in which patient self-determination and autonomy are not generally well-accepted or valued, there could at least be the openness to check and see whether or not an individual patient, in fact, buys into the dominant culture.

In my own teaching, I've been telling physicians more and more, "Look, check in with your patient." It's reasonable to say, "There are some things I would like to share with you. How much do you want to know?" And if a patient says, "You know, doctor, I really don't want you to tell me these things," that would be an unusual patient in our U.S. culture, but by checking in, you know that that patient doesn't want to be told, and then you can say, "Well, how do you want me to make decisions?" The patient might answer, "I want you to talk with my son, and tell him everything." In this country, that would be the exception, but that would be respectful, rather than forcing that person to live by the dominant culture. I don't know why you couldn't do the opposite in other cultures, and simply give the opportunity for the exceptional patient, i.e., the patient who may not share the dominant values, to say, "I do want to make these plans. I do run my life differently."

WHAT TO DO DIFFERENTLY

ALR: *What would you do differently if you were starting Respecting Your Choices™ now?*

BH: I think I'd change the wording of the name of the program (Respecting Your Choices™: An Advance Directive Education Program), by deleting the words "Advance Directive." Instead, I'd want to talk about advance care planning. What we've found is that the words "Advance Directive" always take people back to the document, and the document is just an outcome of the process we're interested in. What is essential is the conversation and all it entails—reflection, understanding, and communicating with loved ones and health care practitioners about values and preferences. Advance care planning and advance directives are not about death, but are about living well near the end of life. You can reformulate advance care planning to focus on the following kinds of questions: How do you want to live when you may be very ill and may not recover? In what way would medicine and medical treatment be helpful? Are there kinds of medical treatment that might interfere with respecting who you are and your dignity? I think grounding the conversation in people's lives puts a slightly different perspective on what we're thinking about. I'd like to see greater focus on what it means to provide good care for someone we love near the end of that person's life. In that way, advance care planning is as much about relationships as it is about values and medical treatment.

> *I think grounding the conversation in people's lives puts a slightly different perspective on what we're thinking about. I'd like to see greater focus on what it means to provide good care for someone we love near the end of that person's life. In that way, advance care planning is as much about relationships as it is about values and medical treatment.*

Interview script

I would like to ask you some questions regarding your views or thoughts about future medical treatment. I know that these questions make some people uneasy, but I want to assure you that we ask all patients these questions. We ask so we might understand and respect your values and beliefs.

Have you ever written down any of your thoughts or choices about future medical treatment, say in a "power of attorney for health care," a living will, or some other type of advance directive? (You might need to explain what each of these names mean. See the definitions at the end of this section.)

If the answer is yes:
Is this document in your medical record?

If the answer is no:
Have you ever considered or thought about these issues for yourself?

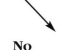

No
Would you like to have it put into your medical record?

Would you like to receive some education materials besides this information card (point out card to patient) or would you like to talk with someone about advance directives? (Check resource list for options.)

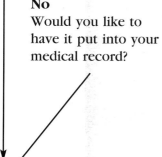

Yes
Would you want anyone to review the document to make sure it is up-to-date?

Is there anything you would like the staff to know about your thoughts or values regarding your medical care?

Protocol

If a patient is too ill or confused at admission, we should ask the above questions later or ask the family if it can provide the answers to the questions.

Reproduced here with permission from Respecting Your Choices,™ La Crosse Area Medical Center's Task Force on Advance Directives: Gundersen Lutheran Health System and Franciscan Skemp HealthCare.

Figure 1.   Protocol for Unit Nurses: Asking Patients About Advance Directives

SUBJECT: Advance Directives   INDEX: GHP-1010
SECTION: General Hospital Policy   PAGE: 1 of 2
ORIGINATOR: Bud Hammes   SUPERCEDES: 04/28/92   DATE: 07/14/94

REVIEW: APPROVED BY:

VICE PRES.(1)   MED. STAFF (N/A)

_____   _____   PRESIDENT_____

_____   _____   VICE PRESIDENT_____

_____   _____   DEPT. HEAD_____

_____   _____   MED. DIRECTOR_____

_____   _____   OTHER_____

DISTRIBUTION: All Dept. ANU Bud Hammes Risk Mgt.

OBJECTIVE:

A. To respect the known wishes of patients who have become incapable of making their health care decisions.

B. To better define the obligations of health care professionals with regard to advance directives.

C. To assure that advance directives are available to physicians in a timely manner.

POLICY:

The desires of an adult patient who is capable of making his or her own health care decisions supercede the effect of an advance directive at all times. If an adult patient is incapable of making his or her health care decisions, then the patient's advance directive is presumed to be valid.

GUIDELINES:

A. Definitions:

1. An adult patient is any person at least 18 years old.

2. An advance directive is any written document representing the wishes and values of an adult, either while a patient or prior to becoming one, that: (a) designates another person(s), i.e., surrogate(s), to make health care decisions on behalf of the patient if the patient is unable to make decisions for himself or herself; (b) gives instructions to a health care professional as to the patient's desires about health care decisions; or (c) both designates a surrogate and gives instructions.

To meet this definition, for the purposes of this policy, an advance directive need not comply with any particular form or formalities, as long as it

Figure 2.   Lutheran Hospital-La Crosse Policy-Procedure Manual

This document comes from the appendix to Chapter 10 of the
Respecting Your Choices™ Training Manual and is not copyrighted.[5]

is in written form and it appears to be authentic. (IT SHOULD BE NOTED THAT ADVANCE DIRECTIVES THAT DO NOT MEET THE STATUTORY RE-QUIREMENTS OF WISCONSIN'S CHAPTER 154 OR 155 MAY NOT PRO-VIDE THE LEGAL PROTECTION AS SPECIFIED IN THOSE STATUTES.)

   3. A primary physician is the attending physician who is responsible for the patient's care.

B. <u>Notification of Entrance or Removal of a Written Advance Directive</u>:

Before an advance directive can be entered into, or removed, from a patient's chart, an authorized staff person from Gundersen Clinic or Lutheran Hospital–La Crosse must be notified. Authorized staff includes: anyone on the medical staff; a patient service representative from Gundersen Clinic; or a person designated by a member of the medical staff who is also either a physician assistant, nurse-practitioner, or a certified advance directive counselor.

The authorized staff [member] must acknowledge notification by making his or her signature on the appropriate line of the patient's advance directive record.

C. <u>Effect</u>:

An advance directive should be followed to the extent that it does not require a physician to perform any act, does not violate that physician's personal or professional ethical responsibilities, or does not violate accepted standards of professional practice. If a physician is unwilling to honor an advance directive because it violates his or her personal ethical beliefs, then transferring the care of the patient to another physician should be discussed with the patient or the patient's surrogate(s).

Advance directives relevant to patient care, e.g., "no resuscitation indicated," will be written by the attending physician on the Hospital order sheets.

D. <u>Validity</u>:

In all cases in which an advance directive is to be disregarded, persuasive and credible evidence must exist that:

   1. the patient was not competent at the time the directive was made;

   2. the directive is a forgery; or

   3. the directive has subsequently been revoked by the patient.

E. <u>Review</u>:

Ordinarily, there should be no need to seek review of the enforceability of an advance directive any more than there ought to be routine review of a patient's oral wishes. However, when doubts or conflicts arise, such as when there is conflict between the advance directive and the wishes of the patient's family, or when there is a substantial doubt as to the authenticity of the advance directive, a consultation should be sent to the Hospital Ethics Committee for its recommendation.

Figure 2.   *Continued*

F. Procedures for Entering and Removing:

A written advance directive will be kept in the front of the patient's active chart in a green plastic folder. The folder will contain a patient's advance directive record that is clearly marked "Advance Directive Record" and the record will have the patient's name, clinic number, and birth date. When a directive is entered the authorized staff who is notified will sign and date the advance directive record. The entrance of the directive will also be noted on the master sheet with the date, the phrase "Advance Directive Entered," and the name of the authorized staff who signed the record. When an advance directive is not personally delivered by the patient, a written confirmation of its entrance into the chart will be sent to the patient.

An advance directive will be removed at the patient's oral or written request. When a directive is removed the authorized staff who is notified will sign and date the advance directive record. The advance directive will be returned to the patient. The patient's written request will remain in the correspondence section of the chart. The removal of the advance directive will be provided to another

1. health care facility if a patient is being transferred to that facility from Lutheran Hospital-La Crosse or,
2. health care facility or physician caring for the patient if requested by the patient or the patient's physician.

The responsibility to transfer advance directives, as described in circumstance 1, will fall to the social worker assigned to the nursing unit caring for the patient.

This should be noted on the master sheet with the date, the phrase "Advance Directive Removed," and the name of the authorized staff who was notified.

G. Transferring Advance Directives:

A copy of an advance directive will be provided to another

1. health care facility if a patient is being transferred to that facility from Lutheran Hospital–La Crosse or,
2. health care facility or physician caring for the patient if requested by the patient or the patient's physician.

The responsibility to transfer advance directives, as described in circumstance 1, will fall to the social worker assigned to the nurisng unit caring for the patient.

H. Questions and Information:

If a patient, family members, or Hospital staff have questions or need information about advance directives, the on-call chaplain will be available to address these questions and needs.

Figure 2. *Continued*

Patient Full Name_____ **Respecting Your Choices™**
Patient ID Number_____ (Keep this form in the Advance DirectiveFolder.)
Patient Birthdate_____

Record of written Advance Directive entered or removed from folder:
For each document list: type of document, date entered or removed, and signature of person entering or removing in spaces below.

	Document 1	**Document 2**	**Document 3**	**Document 4**
Type of Document				
Date entered				
Entered by (signature)				
Date removed				
Removed by (signature)				

Materials Given or Viewed:	**Date:**	**Who was involved in discussion?**
Information Card_____	_____	_____
Booklet_____	_____	_____
Video_____	_____	_____
Worksheet_____	_____	_____
State Document_____	_____	_____

Comments (**with date and signature**)

_____

_____

_____

_____

_____

_____

_____

ADVANCE DIRECTIVES RECORD

Figure 3.   Education Record: Advance Directives Record

This document comes from the appendix to Chapter 10 of the
Respecting Your Choices™ Training Manual and is not copyrighted.[5]

REFERENCES

1. Hammes BJ, Rooney BL. Death and end-of-life planning in one Midwestern community. *Arch Int Med* 1998;158:383–390.
2. Miles SM, Koepp R, Weber EP. Advance end-of-life treatment planning: A research review. *Arch Int Med* 1996;156:1062–1069.
3. The Study to Understand Prognoses and Preferences for Outcomes and Risks of Treatments (SUPPORT). A controlled trial to improve care for seriously ill hospitalized patients. *JAMA* 1995;274:1591–1597.
4. Pearlman RA, Uhlmann RF, Jecker NS. Spousal understanding of patient quality of life: Implications for surrogate decisions. *J Clin Ethics*. 1992;3:114–123.
5. Hammes B, ed. [with contributions from Bernard Hammes, Carol Garman, Nickijo Hager, Elaine Colvin, Dan Felten and Gale Kreibich]. *Respecting Your Choices™ Training Manual*. La Crosse, WI: Lutheran Hospital–La Crosse, 1994, 1996.

International Perspectives

In this section, commentators from Israel, Australia, Spain, Italy, and The Netherlands talk about the use of advance directives—living wills and health care proxies—in their own settings, and, more generally, comment on how end-of-life decision making is approached in their countries. As a group, the commentators eschew the use of formal advance directives and focus, instead, on the central role of communication in establishing and sustaining effective patient–physician relationships. Cultivating such relationships, they assert, is key to providing exemplary end-of-life care.

These perspectives are edited excerpts of interviews conducted with each commentator by Karen S. Heller, PhD, and Anna L. Romer, EdD

The Truth, the Whole Truth, and Nothing But the Truth?

SHIMON GLICK, MD

Ben Gurion University
Beer Sheva, Israel

Living wills (specific treatment-preference documents) have no legal force in Israel at the moment. Some people are pushing for them but, thus far, these documents really have not made much impact. I personally think that such documents are not really the ideal way to go, because it is very hard to predict in advance what a situation is going to be at a given moment. I think designating a proxy, somebody whom one really trusts, makes more sense, although we do not have durable "power of attorney for health care" laws in Israel yet either. We have a patients' rights law, which was enacted in 1996, and the law explicitly outlines what information one has to give a patient. This law clearly stipulates that one must tell the diagnosis, prognosis, alternate forms of therapy, and side effects. If one decides that a patient would be seriously endangered by telling him or her something, then one has to go to an ethics committee to get permission to withhold the information, although in practice I do not know of any doctor who has done that.

CONSTRAINTS ON PATIENT SELF-DETERMINATION

Also, according to Israeli law, there are occasions when one can give a competent patient treatment that he or she is refusing. This is addressed in the law because, before it was written, the question came up: Should one ever force a patient to undergo a life-saving procedure against his or her will? Before the law was passed, the attorney general called a meeting of approximately 30 different people—lawyers, philosophers, rabbis, and doctors—from all over the country, and he asked, "What should we do?" On the one side, were the civil libertarians, who said, "Of course you can't force anybody against his or her will, no matter what." On the other side, were some of the rabbis who spoke of the sanctity of human life. One of the philosophers said, "I have a conflict between my mind and my heart. My mind tells me autonomy, but I can't see a guy lying on the railroad tracks, waiting for the train to come, and not push him off even if he says, 'No.'"

The law, as it was finally written, says essentially: If there is a competent patient, if he or she has been fully informed, if there's a clear-cut danger to his or her life, and he or she could be saved, *and* if an ethics committee has reason to believe that if you force him or her to accept therapy, he or she will subsequently thank you for it, you can do it. Now, when I heard this, I thought it was ridiculous. One would need skills of prophecy. That was my first reaction.

But I shall tell a story: A young Bedouin patient came into one of the big hospitals in Israel. His condition was pneumococcal pneumonia, which was completely treatable. He was having trouble breathing, and the staff wanted to intubate him. He refused, so the resident did not do it, and he died. That is what one would do in any American hospital. Correct? He was alert, he was competent, and he said, "No. I don't want you to intubate me." So, they did not intubate him.

Now this man did not want to die; he was not a cancer patient. He was a young man, he had children. He was afraid, probably. So, after this case, I saw more sense in the Israeli law. He would certainly thank you a hundredfold the next morning, if he had the tube in for 3 or 4 hours and someone had pulled him out of this particular phase of his illness and the antibiotics had taken hold.

In my ward, we applied this law while treating a hunger striker. We fed him under court order. Most Western countries say that it is unethical to do that. The Israeli judge said that, in the conflict between the dignity of the patient and his life, in our society, his life must take precedence. But society in the United States is a different society with different values. I think we have a very strong ethos here supporting the sanctity of life, and still a very strong reaction to the Holocaust.

TRUTH TELLING AND PATERNALISM

There is also a strong paternalistic component to medicine in Israel. Here, the medical establishment basically comes from Europe. Most of the physicians in Israel have not been trained in Israel. So, our foundations of medicine are East European, German, Polish, and Russian, all of which are very paternalistic with very little focus on patient decision making. Also, our system in medical schools was the professorial system, in which the professor is the head of the department; he makes all the decisions; he knows everything. Students have nothing to say about anything, and patients have nothing to say about anything. We are gradually moving over toward a more Western model, but this process is much slower than in the United States. So, I think all of those things put together probably make for a more paternalistic attitude toward patients than in America, although this is changing. There is no question that the whole medical scene, as well as the whole society, is changing. However, those are the components that really make an impact on medicine in Israel today.

There was an article in *Lancet* approximately 7 or 8 years ago that described what doctors tell patients. Researchers took a poll of gastroenterologists at the European gastroenterologic meeting, and it was a dramatic demonstration of different cultural views, because the doctors from the Scandinavian countries invariably told the truth, the doctors from Eastern European countries never told the truth, and the doctors from the Mediterranean countries *almost* never told the truth. The researchers gave seven cases and asked people what they would normally do, and as one went further north, the model resembled the United States model more and more closely.

Now, I came from the United States and have lived half of my professional life there, so I am fairly patient-oriented. However, I am not as great a believer in 100 percent autonomy as many of my American colleagues are. I have seen many situations in which patients defer to the doctor, and prefer the doctor to make the decision for them, and feel more comfortable that way. While I think one should tell

> *While I think one should tell the truth to patients in general, there are times when I do not. I think there are times when patients do not want it and they become very upset when one does tell the truth.*

the truth to patients in general, there are times when I do not. I think there are times when patients do not want it and they become very upset when one does tell the truth.

TREATING EVERY PATIENT INDIVIDUALLY

I think we must treat every patient individually rather than have fixed formulas for everybody. One has to listen to the patient and try to find out what he or she wants to hear. This is not very easy, and we make mistakes. There was a patient on our ward who had metastatic cancer. This man was not told that he had cancer, (allright?). He was in a service that did not tell patients. During a reoccurrence of his disease, he asked the doctor, "Doc, it's what I had last time I have now, right?" He prodded the doctor, asking, "Why don't you tell me?" Finally, he extracted the information from his doctor. But later, during rounds, he chastised his physician, saying, "Doctor, 3 days ago, I asked you how things were with me, how much time do I have to live? You told me that things are not good, they're very bad. That's not a way you should talk to your patients." And he proceeded to give us all a little lecture, as we went past him on rounds.

I was fascinated by this man and asked him if I could interview him, so we could learn more about the best ways to talk with patients. During the interview,

I questioned him, "Why did you ask your doctor to tell you what you had, but when he did, you got angry?"

He said, "It was a stupid question."

"No, no, no," I said. "You're a smart man. Why did you ask that question?"

He said, "I'll tell you why. I wanted him to tell me, 'It's not as bad as you think it is, okay? You can survive.' That's what I wanted him to tell me."

So there's the lesson: the patient knows the truth, he or she wants the truth, but he or she doesn't want the *whole* truth.

Another patient, a Hungarian woman in her 80s, was in the advanced stages of cancer. She was still alert; she was not going to get therapy to cure her. She was going to get supportive therapy, palliative therapy, and she was quite comfortable and quite happy. She did not know she had cancer, and her daughter was adamant that we not tell her. What good would I have done to that patient in the last week of her life to tell her she had cancer, if her daughter was insisting that that was not what she wanted to know?

Advance Care Planning in the Australian Context

LINDA KRISTJANSON, PhD

Edith Cowan University
Perth, Australia

In Australia, a number of the issues around end-of-life decisions, communication, truth telling, family participation in decisions about the goals of care, and advance care planning are addressed in the relationship with the general practitioner (GP), and within the context of the patient receiving palliative care. The GP in Australia is generally more involved in the care experience of patients near the end of life and is more actively integrated into the palliative care service than in the United States. Depending on the region of Australia, between 28 and 70 percent of people who are eligible for palliative care receive it, and the GP is very much a part of that system of care. The majority of palliative care happens at home and is provided by an interdisciplinary team and the home hospice service, which is integrated into the general practice program. There is also a roving, consultative palliative care team in a tertiary care hospital and designated beds in some hospitals as well. But the majority of services occur in the community with the involvement of a GP. What is helpful is that the patient and family usually have a long-term relationship with the GP, with a basis for communication.

Once a person is receiving palliative care, many of the issues involved in end-of-life decisions become almost non-issues. A decision has been made about a type of care and, within that framework of care, those decisions are discussed, and in a sense, people accept that certain things will not happen. It is not necessary to make a fuss about questions such as resuscitation and those kinds of issues. They are taken care of in the move to the palliative care model; it is just part of the ongoing relationship. So, if a patient is ac-

> *Once a person is receiving palliative care, many of the issues involved in end-of-life decisions become almost non-issues. A decision has been made about a type of care and, within that framework of care, those decisions are discussed, and in a sense, people accept that certain things will not happen. It is not necessary to make a fuss about questions such as resuscitation and those kinds of issues. They are taken care of in the move to the palliative care model; it is just part of the ongoing relationship.*

cepted into a palliative care service, there is a clear discussion with the family that resuscitation is not a usual practice (of course, that is different if the patient is also receiving supportive care and symptom management in conjunction with active treatment in another setting). Once that is taken care of, the resuscitation matter dissolves, so to speak. Questions around other aspects of advance directives, about tube-feeding or about the use of intravenous lines or antibiotics, are discussed with the family and the patient as the illness progresses, with the care team trying to stay a little ahead of the family in terms of preparing it and anticipating the kinds of things it may or may not want.

The use of an advance directive in that setting would be inappropriate because it would be seen, as they say here, as "over the top," which means one would not do it; it would not be appropriate. One knows one's patients; the relationship is very individualized. This would be seen as a legalistic kind of document that would be incongruent in the context of the relationship. This might be more appropriate for the younger population who are perhaps healthy, who might be wanting to sort this out with their GPs should they develop illnesses. And that is not the practice here at all.

TRUTH TELLING

In Australia, the diagnosis is clearly disclosed in the majority of cases. Prognosis is discussed in varying degrees of detail, depending on the relationship with the GP and the patient and the family. I think that when the GP maintains control of the care and care is primarily in the home or in the nursing home setting, there is more openness.

In the acute-care setting, it works well when one has a roving palliative care consultative team that is available to anyone in the hospital and can be called in to consult about symptoms, communication issues, and psychological problems. This kind of team seems to act as a catalyst to prompt more truth telling, to encourage more discussion about the actual goals of care, and, often, to facilitate a more appropriate treatment plan; but that depends a lot on the dynamics of the team and the assertiveness of the nurses and other health care professionals to call this team in. One would find this kind of very experienced palliative care consultative team in a large teaching hospital in Australia.

Difficulties with truth telling occur if there is a fast downward illness trajectory, and the patient is receiving care usually within an acute-care hospital that is primarily under the control of a specialist, where the GP may have been marginalized. Then, the specialist is steering the plan of care to a greater extent, and will not be likely to have had a long-term relationship with the patient and family, and will be focusing more on active treatment. The patient moves from active treatment to death. The family has not been prepared and no one has really put this together in a very coordinated way. That is when one sees the difficulties, when there has not been an opportunity to discuss things. The specialist involved is not focusing on that aspect. He or she is focusing on, say, tumor response to the treatment, rather than on larger issues, and sometimes this creates problems for the staff.

So, there are still a number of problems associated with truth telling and "breaking bad news" and a lack of training and education among health professionals and doctors in particular about this whole communication issue. We recently conducted a small Delphi survey of the cancer nurses in the service where I have a consultancy, to identify the key issues related to providing cancer care in an acute care setting. More than half of the concerns relate to communication and palliative care. It comes up again and again, and the nurses feel like—this is a phrase they use—"piggy in the middle," which comes from a little Australian game. The doctor may not be completely open, the nurse is having to negotiate the day-by-day care, and the family is asking questions or the patient is asking questions, and there is a lack of clarity about goals. That is still a difficulty that I think we need to address seriously in terms of education and the comfort of health professionals in being able to talk about this, because even if they know that they should discuss these matters, they do not know how. There are also difficulties with team communication in sorting out the goal of care.

ADVANCE DIRECTIVES AS COMMUNICATION TOOLS

The acute care setting is where a communication tool would be very useful, which is basically what an advance directive is. It is a cue, a way to open the door, a catalyst for opening up discussions about this in a more open way.

One study is underway right now at our institution to examine the use of written advance directives in the nursing home population. In that care setting, when patients and families talk about what they would like in the way of advance directives, 90 percent of them say palliative care. If they become ill, if they become faced with unacceptable illness, if illness debilitates them—that is the route they would want to take. The challenge of implementing this practice is the cost associated with educating all the care providers who may have to act on advance directives. The cost in time associated with working through advance directives with patients and families is seen as quite large. Also, the need to then go out to all the hospitals where a patient might suddenly arrive with one of these on the record and to know what to do with such directives has taken a great deal of money and time.

Some of the families do not think we need to do this degree of serious detailed documentation about advance directives. Other families have found it to be quite helpful, saying, "We've never talked with Mom about this, and we didn't know how to talk with her about it; it's been very helpful." The staff have been quite welcoming of it, once the members understand it, they think that this is a good idea and think maybe they should get advance directives for themselves. People in their 40s and 50s are more receptive to the idea that this might be useful. Older populations tend to say, "Well, my doctor would know best anyway, wouldn't he?" and so they tend to be more passive in the care decision process and are quite trusting. There is not the history of concern about litigation here that you find in the United States.

CULTURALLY APPROPRIATE COMMUNICATION

As the number of new Australians increases, with vastly different cultural and religious backgrounds, communication issues about end-of-life care are a challenge for the staff. The country has been predominantly Christian in terms of religious background. As we have more people come to this country of Muslim background, for instance, it has been a challenge to know with whom to communicate, who the gatekeepers are in terms of information sharing, especially with the patient, how information is shared and communicated, what the gender differences are, and the importance of not taking away hope, which can be a limitation in talking candidly about treatment outcomes. And who controls that communication? These are problems.

We have very, very little information about the Aborigine community, for example. Aborigines who present with cancer do so generally at a much later stage of disease. There are some beginning studies examining beliefs about cancer and palliative care among this group of people. We need to be able to understand these culturally held views. There may be many Aboriginal dialects and languages in one community. At a conference, Deborah Prior from Queensland University in Australia reported that there is no Aboriginal word for "health"; the word that is closest in translation would be "body-spirit-earth." So, the notion of one's own personal health would be a very different concept. The idea of an advance directive to take care of an individual's self-determination needs would be inappropriate. What a person from this cultural background might be more concerned about is the good of the community and that there is probably something out of balance with body, spirit, and the earth and the community. So, the cultural issues about provision of care are really important.

Cultural Attitudes Toward Death and Dying in Spain

JUAN M. NÚÑEZ OLARTE, MD, PhD

Hospital General Universitario Gregorio Marañón
Madrid, Spain

TRUTH TELLING

We have been doing a lot of research on truth telling, and I would say that the picture nowadays in Spain is complex and fluctuating.[1] Society is changing continuously and, on the one hand, we are no longer the Spaniards we used to be 100 years ago, and on the other hand, we are not just part of the "global village." We have to accept that we are simultaneously dealing with different generations and different situations.

What one finds, when summarizing all these data is that, presently, roughly 25 to 50 percent of cancer patients in Spain have their diagnoses disclosed to them. But, if you take suspicion into account, or even what we call *subjective certainty*, this percentage would rise to somewhere between 40 and 70 percent of patients knowing the truth about their conditions. Subjective certainty is a concept we developed based on our research and experience with cancer patients in Spain. It means that the patient knows for sure he or she is going to die, or that he or she has cancer, but no one has told him or her. But this patient knows for sure. He or she does not need anyone to tell him or her, because he or she already knows.

On the other hand, depending on the particular study, somewhere between 16 to 58 percent of patients do not want to have any more information on the true nature of their diseases. In our own study,[2] we found that one third of our patients wanted to know and they knew; one third of the patients did not want to know, and they did not know; and one third were halfway between and they only wanted a little information. But when one is facing death, if one wants a little information, actually, one is saying one does not want information. This third group, then, seems to be a mixture of does-not-want-to-know, but suspects, the truth.

Relatives are also frequently against truth telling. Depending on the study, somewhere between 61 and 73 percent of the families do not want the truth to be disclosed to the patient. Some people describe a "conspiracy of silence," wherein relatives prevent patients from obtaining the truth. But perhaps this is because the families know the patients, and they know the patients do not want to know.

There is a similar problem in interpreting physicians' behavior. In the initial studies, because of the influence of the Anglo-Saxon approach, there was a tendency to look at these figures of a large number of physicians not wanting to disclose the truth as not being in a good direction. At that time, there were no data coming from studies of patients themselves, and so the early researchers were expecting patients to behave the same as they behave in other environments. With the data we have right now, I think it is that the physicians, in a way, are mirroring the population they are taking care of.

Probably, if a physician has been working for a long time, he or she has been exposed to a lot of patients over two or three decades. In the early years, when that physician was shaping an attitude towards truth disclosure, he or she was facing a population in Spain that was even more adamant about not knowing. In fact, that is something that came out also very strongly from a study and was statistically significant: The younger the patient is, the more willing that person is to have information, whereas older patients do not want truth to be disclosed.

"SPANISH DEATH"—ARS MORIENDI

The traditional good death in Spain is what we call "Spanish Death." Spanish Death is the traditional style of death that has been in place in Spain since the 16th and 17th centuries, during the Counter-Reformation. At that time, Spain was a predominantly Catholic country, strongly supporting Counter-Reformation after the Reformation and the birth of Protestant churches in Northern Europe. It was very important at that time to emphasize several aspects when Catholic Spaniards were facing death. Those aspects were basically that death was something very good, not bad . . . one was dying in this life, but one was being born to a much better life, so it was not acceptable that someone would cry or that anyone would react in what we would call nowadays a very human way. This kind of wailing and crying was not acceptable then, but realizing that it was inevitable that a death would have an emotional impact on relatives, the treatises of good dying in Spain emphasized the importance of the relatives not being around. These treatises, called "*ars moriendi*," were very popular.[3]

The physician would come into the room, saying that there was nothing else to be done. Then he or she would retire. Then one would have the priest come and help the dying person to prepare for the impending death. At that time, relatives would have to go out, and then friends would come in, and these friends would have to be Catholic and pious, and they would keep telling the man or the woman that what was going to happen was not bad, but good. We were very, very strongly devoted to this.

Let me illustrate this way. The two kings who have been the most important in the history of Spain were Charles V of Germany and Spain, and Phillip II. Both lived in the 16th century. Both retired prior to their deaths. Charles V did not die a king. He asked his son Phillip II to take the kingdom, and he went into a monastery for seven months to get ready for his death. His son later did the same and died in his bed in his palace, which was built in the monastery.

Just imagine, over the span of 100 years when Spain was the most important country in Western Europe, the two monarchs gave the same message to the kingdom: "You have to get ready." At that time, sudden death, what was called the *"Mors subita et improvisa,"* was really hated. That was the worst death that one could expect, because one was not allowed time enough to get ready for it. So most Spaniards who were literate would carry in their pockets what were called *"Cartas de Aviso."* These "warning letters" were small pieces of paper on which were stamped or painted images depicting death or dying or the saints or the Virgin Mary with admonitions in verses that reminded one of the fleetness of life.

I am not saying that patients who are dying in Spain now are dying the way they were dying in the 17th century—no, not at all. But sometimes, one finds what we call Spanish Death in our elderly patients. We use this term regularly in the unit. When we find one of these patients, and we are discussing in the team how to take care of him or her, we say, "Oh, Señor So-and-So is dying the Spanish Death." That implies a very specific approach we have to take with the patient. These patients come from rural areas; they are not very literate. Each of these patients is probably reenacting the type of death witnessed from the father, who witnessed the grandfather's death, who witnessed the death of the great-grandfather. It probably has nothing to do now with religion, nothing to do with convictions. It is a cultural pattern.

There are some things one has to be very careful about. For these patients, invasive procedures are not acceptable. Just performing a fecal disimpaction might be very stressful. First of all, most of them have *subjective certainty*. They know for sure they're going to die. They do not need anybody telling them so. They know it, and they just want to be left alone. If one is very invasive, either with subcutaneous hydration or fecal disimpaction or any aggressive intervention—I mean, one is missing the point completely.

The other issue is that they don't want their families around. There is nothing special about it, it is just that that is the way they think it has to be done. On the one hand, it is intrusive on their own privacy, because they want to be left alone. And, most of the time, they take fetal positions, they face the windows, with their backs toward the door. It is very simple; the message is that they are receding.

This can be very upsetting to relatives. Most of the time, they do not know why this kind gentleman or kind lady, who has been so kind and gracious for most of his or her life, in the last days of living just does not want to communicate. And I keep telling them, these patients are dying the way they think they should die. It is putting a very stoic face on it.

If one does not explain this to the family members, they feel guilty. They feel there is something missing and that they are being punished because something has been wrong. So, it is very interesting because, actually, the elderly are dying in a cultural environment that is old like they are, whereas the younger generations do not understand the behavior, and one has to explain what is going on.

ADVANCE DIRECTIVES HAVE "GONE NOWHERE" IN SPAIN

In the early 1990s, when the palliative care movement started, there was very strong support for advance directives by the Catholic Church and a lot of other organizations, taking them straight from the American model. But the idea has simply gone nowhere. In our own practice, the largest palliative care unit in Spain, we take care of more than 1000 new patients per year. I have not seen one single advance directive in eight years.

The American model puts a lot of attention on autonomy, empowering the patient, and I think that is the right way to go and that is the way we are going now in Spain. But that does not mean throwing autonomy on top of people. Autonomy does not mean assaulting them with truth, or assaulting them with informed consent, or assaulting them with advance directives.

Also, we change styles of living during our lives. We change marriages. We change political sides. We change religious convictions. When we are facing death, are we not going to change? I am not at all interested in what people are saying when they are healthy. I want to know what people think when they are facing death. Instead of advance directives, one has to understand what people want at that time.

It requires that one always be sensitive enough to realize what type of patient one is facing. If one is facing a traditional style of patient, then one has to be a paternalistic physician in a way. These patients do not want to make decisions. And if one tries to push them to make decisions, one put them into anguish, one builds a lot of anxiety, both in the patient and in the family, because that is not what they want from their doctors. They want the doctor to make the decisions for them. One has to realize whether the patient is this type "A" or if the patient is type "C." Type C is a young patient with a different approach, who really wants to be informed and really wants to share all the decision process, and wants to choose the different therapeutic options, even to the very last. But, most of the time, these patients want to choose when there are cure-oriented treatment options. They do not want to choose so much when the treatment is just palliative. One is not choosing how to live, but how to die. Then one has the "type B" patient, which is the patient that does not know he or she is dying, but suspects it, and is caught in between. I

> We change styles of living during our lives. We change marriages. We change political sides. We change religious convictions. When we are facing death, are we not going to change? I am not at all interested in what people are saying when they are healthy. I want to know what people think when they are facing death.

would say that the vast majority of our patients are B types. It is neither a question of white nor black; it is gray—different shades of gray.

There is an artistic part to doing palliative care in Spain. One has to have a lot of skills in order to face the patient, to probe, to understand how much does he or she want to know? If one has a patient that does not want to be informed at all, or very little, then one has to figure out what the approach is towards certain treatments without actually telling the truth. This is something that is better witnessed than explained. If one comes to our unit, or to any unit in Spain, and just watches physicians doing that, one would realize immediately that we are talking about this without talking about it. There is a lot of nonverbal communication.

DEFAULT POSITION ON RESUSCITATION IN SPANISH HOSPITALS

In most palliative care units, it is understood that if there is a cardiac arrest, there is not going to be any resuscitation attempt. That is understood by all professionals, but there are relatives who do not want to understand that. This is not an easy conversation for any Spanish relative. It is like trying to get permission from a relative to perform an autopsy. It is very seldom we get autopsies in palliative care units in Spain, because most of the relatives feel that the doctor is adding the last straw to the haystack and they do not want to take it. It is the last aggression. Even though the patient is already dead, they do not want it.

Relatives are not involved in discussions about resuscitation. It is not a concern of patients, nor of families. They are concerned about whether the patient is going to suffer. They are concerned about whether the patient is going to be lucid or not. But they are not involved in resuscitation discussions.

REFERENCES

1. Centeno Cortes C, Núñez Olarte JM. Estudios sobre la cómunicación del diagnóstico de cáncer en España. *Med Clin (Barc)* 1998;110:744-750.
2. Centeno Cortes C, Núñez Olarte JM. Questioning diagnosis disclosure in terminal cancer patients: A prospective study evaluating patients' responses. *Palliat Med* 1994;8:39-44.
3. Fernández-Shaw Toda M. Ars moriendi: Images of death in Spanish art. *Eur J Palliative Care* 1997;4:164-168.

Speaking in a Particular Way: Individualizing Communication for Each Patient

CARLA RIPAMONTI, MD

National Cancer Institute
Milan, Italy

In Italy, we do not have advance directives; it is not a concept for us. We also have no Do-Not-Resuscitate orders in our clinical charts. We think it is awkward to ask patients too far in advance about whether they would want to be resuscitated. It would depend, would it not, on the circumstances? Because every patient, even if at the very end of life, is different. A patient with good pain control and good family support is different from a patient whose pain we have been unable to control, or who is suffering from very severe dyspnea or from severe psychological distress. One would not resuscitate a patient with very severe dyspnea, but if one had a patient also in the terminal stages of illness but with a very good quality of life, one might try resuscitation if the patient wanted to be resuscitated. It is necessary to consider each patient as an individual.

AN INDIVIDUAL APPROACH

The question is: Will the treatment bring a benefit to the patient? In Italy, the doctor has the authority to make that decision and so, for this reason, the doctor carries a great deal of responsibility. However, certainly, at our institution, it is often a collaborative decision in which physicians talk with patients and families. It happens within the relationship between the doctor and the patient.

Here at the National Cancer Institute of Milan and, in particular, in our division of palliative care, communication is considered a very important part of the treat-

> *I think it is important to communicate everything to the patient, but it is important to consider the way you communicate. We have some patients who want to know their situations exactly and explicitly, so we speak precisely with them. And we give all our patients the opportunity to ask everything. We try to understand what, and how much, they want to know.*

ment, of the cure, and of the care. One must spend time with patients to understand their needs. How else could one tell if the pain was a physical pain or a psychological pain? Only by talking with the patient, can one decide whether to increase the dose of morphine or provide more psychological support.

We speak continuously with patients and their families. Some patients tell us, for example, "Don't prolong my life." Or, "I need to live one more month because I need to see my son." Patients and families and their doctors talk together about what would be the best thing to do. We have a very personal approach, with different goals for each patient.

TRUTH TELLING

Unfortunately, there is not such good communication and discussion with patients and families throughout Italy. In many parts of the country, one will find that doctors do not communicate the diagnosis of cancer to their patients, and they may not have good communication with the family at all. Sometimes patients are treated with chemotherapy without knowing that it is chemotherapy. It is not possible to say this word, "cancer," because in Italy, cancer is associated with great suffering. So it is rather difficult for the doctor to use this word and for the patient to accept it without explaining that there exists the possibility to cure the cancer and to care for the patient throughout his or her illness. Perhaps as we palliative care specialists get better at doing this—letting families and doctors know that cancer does not have to mean suffering, that it is possible to have pain control, to die among family and friends in comfort—perhaps then the word "cancer" will create fewer problems.

But right now, it is often much more acceptable to speak about death than to speak about cancer. To have a cancer is something terrible, while death is part of one's destiny. Yet even so, after 15 years of working with cancer patients, I have never said to a patient "you are dying," unless specifically requested to do so by the patient.

I also think that awareness of prognosis or of impending death differs day by day. One could have a patient who clearly knows his or her prognosis, but when he or she feels better he or she believes that death is not near. One day we are able to accept death; the day after, we are not.

One must use appropriate words. For example, I say: "The illness is very serious, but we can try to control your pain and other symptoms; I will not leave you alone, and I will do everything to improve the quality of your life, but your illness is very serious."

I think it is important to communicate everything to the patient, but it is important to consider the *way* you communicate. We have some patients who want to know their situations exactly and explicitly, so we speak precisely with them. And we give all our patients the opportunity to ask everything. We try to understand what, and how much, they want to know.

I also think that awareness of prognosis or of impending death differs day by day. One could have a patient who clearly knows his or her prognosis, but when he or she feels better he or she believes that death is not near. One day we are able to accept death; the day after, we are not.

Many families worry that their loved ones will not ever be able to accept the truth. Sometimes a family member will take the physician aside and say, "Please do not give the prognosis to my parent or to my son or my mother. He will commit suicide if he knows everything, or she will grow despondent." In these cases, we see the family as our patient too, and we must give it support. Our home care program has been very helpful in situations like this. When nurses, doctors, and volunteers go into a patient's home, they can see how the family is organized; they can help the family each moment the patient is alive. It is important to support the family and to help the family realize that it is important to say what is happening, but one must do so in a *particular* way.

THE PATIENT ARRIVES AT HIS OR HER OWN PROGNOSIS

The patient must be the real guide. For example, when I have to say that the prognosis is not good and that the illness is worsening, I speak with the patient, and I ask him or her to speak about the illness. Through our conversation, he or she arrives at his or her own sense of the prognosis.

For example, I may speak about the sites of the metastases or the fact that the tumor is growing. If the patient then says, "So my health is worsening," I concur. I will reply, "Yes, it is worsening." Through our dialogue, the patient arrives at his or her own prognosis. And one can see this happening. "Is it time for me to call my son in America?" a patient may ask. Or, "Is it better that I stop working? Should I ask for financial support?" In this way, the patient arrives at his or her own prognosis in a way that he or she can comprehend and accept.

After all, none of us can say exactly what will happen. We had some patients come from the United States and Australia and they had been told that they had only 6 months to live. They spent the last months of their lives in a terrible state, sure that they would die at any moment. It would have been better to say that we do not know with certainty when this will happen, but that the disease is very, very serious and that there is no more point to continuing the chemotherapy and the radiotherapy. We must continue with palliative medicine, we must continue with our presence, with home care, with a personal, empathetic involvement, but no more chemotherapy or radiotherapy. So, we speak quite clearly about the need to stop anticancer therapy, we are clear about the seriousness of the illness, without literally saying, "You are dying."

Limitations to Advance Directives: A Dutch View

ZBIGNIEW ZYLICZ, MD, PhD

Hospice Rozenheuvel
Rozendaal, The Netherlands

In The Netherlands, we are not so focused on advance care planning. People do sign advance directives, but they are not fully "waterproof." In other words, doctors are not required to comply with them. I believe that these documents, as I have seen them used, are of no value. One of the problems is that patients create and sign living wills when they are healthy. For us, it is important to find out what the patient wants at the moment when he or she is very ill.

Here is an example from my own experience some time ago: I had a patient, with septicemia and an infection in his bladder, who needed to be resuscitated, but he had an advance directive indicating he did not want to be resuscitated. His family came after the ambulance, saying, "Please do not resuscitate him." I did not comply with their wishes. I did resuscitate him and then moved him to the intensive care unit. Twenty-four hours later, he recovered. When I asked him later about his advance directive, which indicated he did not want to be resuscitated, he said, "I never meant it for this kind of situation." Doctors in The Netherlands still have the privilege and the autonomy to decide what to do at the moment. The law and public feeling are behind them.

We are not under as much legal pressure here as in the United States, and there is more public trust. Patients are increasingly able to complain about services they receive, but getting money from malpractice suits is unusual. We like our patients to be able to complain and we try to be open and frank, but we do not resort to the legal system to resolve differences.

For these reasons, I feel that advance directives, especially specific treatment requests, are not so useful.

RELATIONSHIPS ARE MORE IMPORTANT

Almost half (46 percent) of Dutch people are dying at home, cared for by their general practitioners. Of the remainder, 17 percent are dying in nursing homes and 37 percent in hospitals where they are cared for by nursing home physicians and specialists, respectively. Before palliative medicine was practiced in The Netherlands, patients with complicated terminal illnesses were nursed in hospitals. However, hospitals have 20 percent fewer beds now as compared to 15 years ago and many patients are discharged to home or to nursing homes where there are long waiting lists.

For these reasons, much end-of-life care is provided by GPs and district nurses. These physicians and nurses are the most important part of the health care system for these dying patients and their families. These doctors and nurses visit approximately half of their patients at home and see the other half in the office. The family doctor knows each patient's priorities and ways of coping and can be an important source of information. Older people live in the same communities and have the same doctors for 20 years. Their physicians rely on this long-standing relationship and knowledge. This long-term contact among the patient, the family, the nurse, and the doctor is one of the strongest parts in The Netherlands' medical care. The patient knows the doctor; the doctor is well paid and is someone who is trusted by the whole family. One cannot see communication separately from the system.

Of course, one disadvantage of our system is that many GPs are working alone, in isolation from other colleagues and specialists. That is why a major part of what our hospice does, in addition to the acute care inpatient unit we run, is to provide advice and support to GPs in the community.

Isolation is particularly a problem when it comes to euthanasia. Euthanasia in The Netherlands is decriminalized, but it is not legal. In these situations, very often there is one family and one physician, and they must make the decision alone. The doctor can be very attached to the situation and perhaps could benefit from having the opportunity to talk the situation over with other colleagues. Or, maybe the physician needs more skills in pain and symptom management or how to deal with depression. Our hospice tries to deal with this problem of isolation by providing help with pain and symptom management and being available as a backup for the GP.

INNOVATION IN THE DUTCH CONTEXT

> *In our experience, 80 percent of our patients who request euthanasia are afraid of something—afraid of losing dignity, of being damaged—and their requests for euthanasia come out of fear. When you provide these patients with a safe environment, then, they say three days later, "Doctor this is exactly what I meant." Often, once they feel safe, patients never discuss euthanasia again.*

An innovation in this country would be to introduce the perspective of palliative care, so as to have an alternative to offer people who request euthanasia. Often these people are suffering from hopelessness. Palliative medicine would provide an alternate way of dealing with this hopelessness. I believe that good palliative care would change a lot of requests. I am very liberal about all this. I agree that people must be free to decide about life and death, but it is not moral to offer only one choice; with palliative care, one has more choices.

In our experience, 80 percent of our patients who request euthanasia are afraid of something—afraid of losing dignity, of being damaged—and their requests for euthanasia come out of fear. When you provide these patients with a safe environment, then, they say three days later, "Doctor this is exactly what I meant." Often, once they feel safe, patients never discuss euthanasia again.

Therefore, we must focus on quality of life. We need to bring attention to the patient's quality of life as early as possible. Half of what we are doing in palliative care is prevention, prevention of loss. You can do many things to a patient, for example, control pain, but as a consequence cause loss of ability to drive a car. In that case, the patient has no pain but cannot drive a car to visit his or her daughter. In my opinion, you cannot start palliative care soon enough, and this will require talking with patients about what losses they are willing to accept and what losses the patients want to prevent. The patients should set the agendas.

BARRIERS TO PALLIATIVE CARE

One major barrier to offering best palliative care in The Netherlands is a lack of financing. Enthusiastic doctors, charity money, and foundations have been supporting this work, and now palliative care is beginning to be officially recognized, but it is still a long process. In order to try to translate palliative care into mainstream medicine, we need to have financing. Under the Dutch national health system, people have 100 percent coverage, including terminal care but, in fact, terminal care is not getting reimbursed. On paper, this insurance includes birth to death, but because of a shortage of resources and because of the way money and resources are divided, there is an enormous shortage of money.

OPPORTUNITIES FOR IMPROVEMENT

Up until now, the approach to cancer treatment has been a curative focus—treatment, treatment, treatment. As the numbers of aging and frail people increase, we will have increasing numbers of dying patients, and their families will ask for better care. In addition, I have noticed a change in physicians' attitudes since my training. Medicine in The Netherlands was dominated by men; it was a masculine world. This is now changing rapidly as we have half men and half women in medical school. I see an enormous change because women have a completely different perspective; they attend to the quality of patients' lives. They are not so hard and mindless in their approach to medicine!

Selected Bibliography

Part Two

Articles by contributors to this part:

Centeno Cortés C, Núñez Olarte JM. Questioning diagnosis disclosure in terminal cancer patients: A prospective study evaluating patients' responses. *Palliative Med* 1994; 8:39–44.

Colvin E, Hammes BJ. If I only knew: A patient education program on advance directives. *Am Nephrol Nurs Assn J* 1991;18:557–560.

Hammes BJ, Bottner W, Lapham C. Expanding frames . . . opening choices: Reconsidering conversations about medical care when cure is not possible. *Illness, Crisis, and Loss* 1998;6(4):352–356.

Hammes BJ, Kane RS. CPR practices in Wisconsin long-term care facilities. *WMJ* 1998; 97:55–57.

Hammes BJ, Rooney BL. Death and end-of-life planning in one midwestern community. *Archives of Internal Medicine.* 1998; 58:383–390.

Núñez Olarte JM. Care of the dying in 18th century Spain—the non-hospice tradition. *Eur J Palliative Care* 1999;6(1):23–27.

Núñez Olarte JM, Gracia Guillén D. Cultural issues and ethical dilemmas in palliative and end-of-life care in Spain. *Cancer Control* (in press).

Núñez Olarte JM, Centeno Cortés C. Truth telling: The hispanic perspective. In: Portenoy RK and Bruera E (eds). *Topics in Palliative Care.* Oxford: Oxford University Press (in press).

Solomon MZ, et al. 1997. Advance Care Planning. In: *Decisions Near the End of Life*: Annotated Bibliographies on 10 Topics in End-of-Life Care. Newton, MA: Education Development Center, Inc.

Other selected literature:

Annunziata MA. Ethics of relationship: From communication to conversation. *Ann NY Acad Sci* 1997;809:400–410.

Barrett B, Shadick K, Schilling R, Spencer L, del Rosario S, Moua K, Vang M. H'mong/medicine interactions: Improving cross-cultural health care. *Family Med* 1998;30(3):179–184.

Blackhall L, Murphy, S, Frank, G, Michel V, Azen, S. Ethnicity and attitudes toward patient autonomy. *JAMA* 1995;274 (10): 820–825.

Buckman, R. *How to Break Bad News: A Guide for Health Care Professionals.* Baltimore: The Johns Hopkins University Press, 1992.

Cultural issues in palliative care. (Ch. 10). In: Doyle D, Hanks GWC, MacDonald N, eds. *Oxford Textbook of Palliative Medicine.* Oxford, UK: Oxford University Press, 1998, pp. 777–801.

Ersk M, Kagawa-Singer M, Barnes D, Blackhall L, Koenig BA. Multicultural considerations in the use of advance directives. *Oncol Nurs Forum* 1998;25(10): 1683-1690.

Faulkner A. ABC of palliative care: Communication with patients, families, and other professionals. *Br Med J* 1998:316:130-132.

Fernández-Shaw Toda M. Ars moriendi: Images of death in Spanish art. *Eur J Palliative Care* 1997;4(5):164-168.

Freedman B. Offering truth: One ethical approach to the uninformed cancer patient. *Arch Int Med* 1993;153(5):572-526.

Gordon DR. Disclosure practices and cultural narratives: Understanding concealment and silence around cancer in Tuscany, Italy [review]. *Soc Sci Med* 1997;44(10):1433-1452.

Koenig BA. Cultural diversity in decisionmaking about care at the end of life. In: Field MK, Cassel CK, eds. *Approaching Death: Improving Care at the End of Life*. Washington, DC: National Academy Press, 1997, pp. 363-382.

Koenig B, Gates-Williams J. Understanding cultural difference in caring for dying patients. *Western J Med* 1995;163(3):244-249.

Miles SH, Koepp R, Weber EP. Advance end-of-life treatment planning: A research review. *Arch Int Med* 1996;156:1062-1068.

Sehgal AR, Weisheit C, Miura Y, Butzlaff M, Kielstein R, Taguchi Y. Advance directives and withdrawal of dialysis in the United States, Germany, and Japan. *JAMA* 1996;276(20):1652-1656.

Surbone A. Truth telling to the patient. [letter from Italy]. *JAMA* 1992;268(13): 1661-1662.

Teno JM, Lynn J. Putting advance care planning into action. *J Clin Ethics* 1996;7: 205-214.

Thomsen OO, Wulff HR, Alessandro M, et al. What do gastroenterologists in Europe tell cancer patients? *Lancet* 1993;341(8843):473-476.

Voltz R, Akabayashi A, Reese C, Ohi G, Sass H-M. End-of-life decisions and advance directives in palliative care: A cross-cultural survey of patients and health-care professionals. *J Pain and Symptom Management* 1998;16:153-162.

Part Three

Moving Toward Family-Centered Care

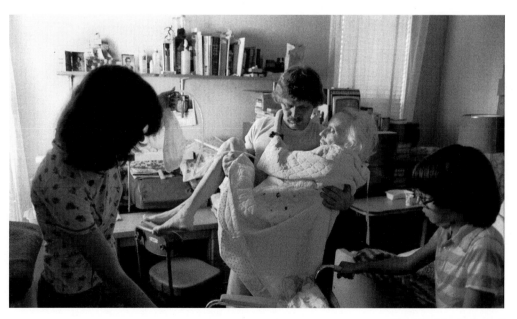

Photo by John Seakwood

Listening to Patients and Families Moves Practice Toward Family-Centered Care

ANNA L. ROMER, EdD

*Education Development Center, Inc.
Newton, Massachusetts*

In the second part of this book, our international editors described how decisions about using or forgoing life-sustaining treatment are made in Israel, Australia, Italy, Spain, and The Netherlands. As Mildred Solomon pointed out in her accompanying editorial, these descriptions revealed a more subtle interpretation of the concept of autonomy. In these countries, the focus seems to be on relationship building, both with individual patients and with their families. There is less interest in trying to document ahead of time, precisely what patients think they will want under unknown future circumstances and more interest in understanding who the patient is, and what he or she wants in the present moment.

In this part we offer a range of pieces that extend this critique. Each of the innovators whose work we present has chosen to listen to patients and families carefully. In so doing, each has developed a more sophisticated understanding of autonomy, which moves us towards legitimizing a more family-centered ethic of care.

Navah Harlow, MA, director of the Center for Ethics in Medicine at Beth Israel Medical Center in New York City, describes a process for bringing families, particularly those from minority cultural groups, back into the decision-making process when their loved ones have lost their own decision-making capacity. Ms. Harlow developed a process of family letter writing, which has enabled families to communicate what they know of the patient's values, beliefs, and wishes in their own words and often in their own languages. These letters are used to help the family clarify its own understanding, and to honor and respect what it knows the patient would want. Because of the idiosyncrasies of New York State law, which requires "clear and convincing evidence" before life support can be withdrawn, hospital ethics committees are where decisions about withdrawing treatment are often taken if patients have left no prior directives about their wishes. Ms. Harlow has used these letters to present the family's case to hospital ethics committees engaged in such deliberation.

Stuart Farber, MD, and his colleagues at Multicare Regional Cancer Center in

Tacoma, Washington, are developing a workbook for patients and families to be used once a cancer diagnosis has been established. As with Navah Harlow's innovation, the purpose of the Farber workbook is to put patients and families back in the "driver's seat" in terms of decision making and informing their clinicians about who they are and how they want to proceed. What is distinctive about this project is that Dr. Farber and his colleagues are attempting to treat the *family* as the unit of care and to do so early on, as soon as the family has learned of the patient's diagnosis. Dr. Farber's interest in this approach was stimulated by focus-group research he conducted with surviving family caregivers. Taking family experiences as the starting point, he and his colleagues came to the same insight suggested by the research on cultural diversity in end-of-life decision making: There are serious limits to assuming patients make decisions autonomously and out of the context of family, culture, community, and the particulars of a given situation.[1-4] When it comes to life-and-death issues, patients and families *together* need to be the unit of care.

> *There are serious limits to assuming patients make decisions autonomously and out of the context of family, culture, community, and the particulars of a given situation. When it comes to life-and-death issues, patients and families together need to be the unit of care.*

In the International Perspectives section of Part Three, two American physicians describe the crosscultural research they have done with patients, families, and physicians around end-of-life issues. These two commentators share how their respective research has challenged their own thinking. Dr. Leslie J. Blackhall describes the ways in which her research into the attitudes and beliefs of patients who were not white middle-class professionals like herself, led her to develop a more subtle concept of autonomy. Really listening to the voices of her informants and going back to ask for clarification about their attitudes led her to discover the coherence in their stories and to reframe what she had initially seen as contradictory attitudes. Dr. Michael D. Fetters, a family physician and researcher who has lived in Japan and studied how Japanese physicians work with patients and families around the question of disclosure of cancer diagnoses, reflects on what his research has taught him. He then shares a real-life example from his practice with Japanese expatriates in Ann Arbor, Michigan.

Family-centered care is a concept that has come out of pediatric literature and practice, but has not yet been widely translated into the care of adults.[5] Attention to issues of cultural diversity and attempts to learn from patients and families from ethnic groups other than white, middle-class Americans highlight the need for expanding current notions of patient-centered care to include the patient's family, however he or she chooses to define "family." Taking questions of diversity seriously allows "mainstream" bioethics to ground theories in lived experience and to interpret and understand principles such as autonomy, in more nuanced ways. Although derived from research on cultural diversity, increased attention to the importance of family is likely to benefit all patients and families, regardless of their ethnic and cultural backgrounds.

REFERENCES

1. Blackhall L, Murphy S, Frank G, Michael V, Azen S. Ethnicity and attitudes toward patient autonomy. *JAMA* 1995;274 (10):820–825.
2. Ersk M, Kagawa-Singer M, Barnes D, Blackhall L, Koenig BA. Multicultural considerations in the use of advance directives. *Oncol Nurs Forum* 1998;25 (10):1683–1690.
3. Koenig BA. Cultural diversity in decisionmaking about care at the end of life. In: *Approaching Death: Improving Care at the End of Life*. Field M, Cassel C, eds. Washington, DC: National Academy Press, 1997, pp. 363–382.
4. Fetters MD. The family in medical decision making: Japanese perspectives. *J Clin Ethics* 1998;(9):132–146.
5. Hostler SL, ed. *Family-Centered Care: An Approach to Implementation.* Charlottesville, VA: University of Virginia, Children's Medical Center, Kluge Children's Rehabilitation Center, 1994.

Family Letter Writing

An Interview with NAVAH HARLOW, MA

Beth Israel Medical Center
New York, New York

New York State law regarding family authority to withdraw life support is more restrictive than that in most states. Families do not have decision-making authority unless they have been appointed as health care agents or unless they have "clear and convincing evidence" of the wishes the patient expressed before the patient lost decision-making capacity. Clinicians at Beth Israel Medical Center, were concerned that this legal framework, grounded in the assumption of the primacy of patient autonomy as the guiding ethical principle, resulted in families, particularly families from distinct minority cultural groups, becoming frustrated that their wishes for the patients and their knowledge of what the patients would want were not being taken into consideration. With the support of upper-level management (the president of the medical center and senior vice president of legal affairs), Navah Harlow, MA., director of the Center for Ethics in Medicine at Beth Israel Medical Center, created a process whereby families could communicate what they knew of each patient's values, beliefs and wishes, so that they could present their cases to the ethics committee in order to honor and respect what they believed the patients would want. What follows are edited comments from an interview with Ms. Harlow by Anna L. Romer, EdD.

I have meetings with families when there is no written advance directive and, sometimes, when I think there might be conflict among family members. Most of the time these conversations are triggered by the necessity of a treatment decision, or by families saying, "Take her off that machine." In these meetings, I ask families the following kinds of questions:

- Tell us who our patient is.
- What kind of a person is your mother?
- You're asking us to withdraw life support; is this what she would want? Tell us how you know.
- Did you ever have an experience in which she commented on another person's situation, when the other person was incapacitated and on life support? Did she relate those experiences to her own personal views for herself?

These questions then lead to wonderful conversations, sometimes very tearful ones, and often, emotional and cathartic moments for families. Once these conversations take place, we have a sense of the patient's own values and preferences and the world view and family values that have guided the patient's life.

I then ask the family to write a letter to me, Navah Harlow, and explain that this letter will be brought before the ethics committee. Because of the strictness of New York State law regarding withdrawal of life support for any patient without a written advance directive, we need to bring the request before an ethics committee before we can remove life support. We are committed to every patient's right to self-determination and so, we offer families this opportunity to honor their loved ones by bringing clear and convincing evidence of their wishes, even though these patients did not articulate them in writing.

These questions then lead to wonderful conversations, sometimes very tearful ones, and often, emotional and cathartic moments for families. The process allows them to clarify and review their loved one's life and helps them articulate what was meaningful for that person. For some family members, this activity of reclaiming the personhood of the patient is experienced as a last act of commitment and caring toward their loved one.

We ask that the family write a letter that includes vignettes that illustrate the patient's values and beliefs (see box Sample Letter). This is a personal letter, not a legalistic one. The patient's family members use their own words to recreate and reflect their loved one's personhood. The family may bring it back the next day or the same day. This letter can be written by one family spokesperson or can be the work of multiple family members, as long as each member signs it and designates his or her relationship to the patient. It can be written in English or in the native tongue of the family. These letters are then used to meet the standard of clear and convincing evidence about the wishes of the patient.

This process seems to be a spiritual one that can bring families closer together. We use this same process even when a written advance directive is in place, if there seems to be hesitation or differences of opinion among family members. The process allows them to clarify and review their loved one's life and helps them articulate what was meaningful for that person. For some family members, this activity of reclaiming the personhood of the patient is experienced as a last act of commitment and caring toward their loved one.

Sample Letter

Ms. Harlow has provided us with the following letter written to her by a family as part of the process of establishing clear and convincing evidence of a patient's wishes. The letter has been edited to exclude identifying information and was translated from its original version in Spanish.

Dear Ms. Harlow:

.........., a good husband, father of ten children, seventy three years old, has dedicated his entire life to his family and his work. An exemplary man to all who knew him, all of his life he has been a solid and healthy person, free-spirited and very active. His sole purpose was to ensure that his family had a healthy environment and a good education.

He arrived in New York in 1983, where he had an unforgettable experience: He saw his grandchild dying while being maintained on a respirator, being kept alive by a machine. He said, "If, someday, this should ever happen to me, never put me on a life-support machine. I believe it is unnecessary suffering to continue someone's life who will not have a complete recovery, who will not ever lead a normal life again." His wife and all his children, knowing his thoughts about this subject, request that you please respect his wishes. Knowing what his current physical condition is, we believe it is inhumane to have us witness our father going through something we know he does not want. We attest to this request with the signatures of his wife and children below.

Living with a Serious Illness:
A Workbook for Patients and Families

An Interview with STUART FARBER, MD

Multicare Regional Center
Tacoma, Washington

In 1997, Stuart Farber, MD, and a team of colleagues at Multicare Regional Cancer Center in Tacoma, Washington, participated in a conference entitled Decisions Near the End of Life: Focus on Cancer Care, a national initiative to improve terminal and palliative care for cancer patients and their families.* His multidisciplinary team became the nucleus of a Decisions Task Force at their hospital, a group of professionals committed to improving care for patients who are facing life-threatening illness and their families. The task force has focused on two main projects: improving pain management (which Dr. Farber reported in 1998 in the Journal of Palliative Medicine,[1]*) and developing a workbook designed to help patients and families who are facing serious illness clarify their own values and goals of care and communicate these effectively to their health care providers. In the following interview with Karen S. Heller, PhD, Dr. Farber describes the steps he and his colleagues on the Decisions Task Force are taking to develop the workbook, and to train health care providers at the Cancer Center to use the information the workbook, provides to improve the quality and continuity of care, communication, and decision making throughout the patient's illness trajectory. Dr. Farber's coinnovators, members of the original core Decisions group, included Bev Hatter, MSW; Linda O'Reiley, RN; Cherie Braden, RN; Lu Farber, MBA; and Kay Lanier, RN.*

Karen S. Heller: *What led you and your colleagues to develop a workbook for patients and families facing serious illness?*

Stuart Farber: It started with a core group, which we called the Decisions Task Force because it coalesced following the participation of a team from our hospital in the Decisions Near the End of Life conference.* The task force originally was composed of six to eight people, including myself. I was the hospice med-

---

*Decisions Near the End of Life: Focus on Cancer Care is an initiative of Education Development Center, Inc., a private not-for-profit research and development organization in Newton, Massachusetts. This national initiative, made possible through a grant from the Open Society Institute's Project on Death in America, is designed to improve terminal and palliative care for cancer patients and their families. The first training conference, held in Destin, Florida in January 1997, was attended by multidisciplinary teams from nineteen comprehensive and community cancer centers from around the United States.

ical director for our health system and the lone "physician champion" on the task force. The group also included the nurse manager of the inpatient oncology unit at the Cancer Center (who has since been promoted to director of the Cancer Center, which has been very helpful to our overcoming barriers to the project) and the nurse manager of the medicine ward at a smaller community hospital in our system, which is a referral hospital to the Cancer Center. We also had a nurse from one of the outpatient oncology clinics, a pharmacist, and one of the managers of the hospice program.

That initial group was important because it represented many different points of view as well as most of the leverage points of where this care is delivered in our system. The group recognized that, despite a lot of very talented people in our hospital system who were dedicated to improving end-of-life care, we just weren't caring for dying patients as well as we could be. So, we asked, "Well, are there other ways to do it?"

As we began to consider how could we do it differently, we discussed where we ourselves had gained our knowledge about caring for patients with serious illness. We realized that, mostly, we learned this from the patients and families whom we cared for and, to some degree, from superlative caregivers at the bedside, both professional and nonprofessional. So, we thought we probably could learn something by talking to the patients and families about their experiences. Listening to what they had to say might give us new insights and information that might lead us to figure out better ways to help patients and families and empower them to take more control over their care, as well as helping us identify leverage points where we could influence providers. We hoped to learn what was good and bad within our system and how we, as a system, might better support both the providers and the patients.

LISTENING TO RECENTLY BEREAVED FAMILY CAREGIVERS

We decided to hold some focus groups. It was not easy to decide to whom we should talk. You want to talk to people who are dying, but that's a very hard thing to do for various reasons. First, they're sick and vulnerable, and it can be a significant burden to try to talk to people while they're going through any number of treatments and vicissitudes of their illnesses. Plus, it's very distracting and, while they're going through this, only a very few people would be able to provide the information. It would be hard to get them together; it would be incredibly labor intensive.

So even though we thought that speaking with patients was a good idea, we abandoned it in favor of talking to the survivors, those family and community members who have cared for people who died. Survivors are a fairly easy group to get together. In general, most people are eager to talk about their experiences, and they're still processing this themselves. So, we went to a contact person in the inpatient, outpatient, and hospice settings in our health system and asked each, "Can you get up to ten people together to have a focus group?" We asked one of the counselors who does social work and counseling support on the inpatient oncology ward, and one of the outpatient nurses, who delivers chemotherapy and supports patients and families, and the bereavement coordinator for the hospice program. Each agreed.

We convened three groups, each averaging eight participants. Most were spouses of cancer patients who had died, but there were also adult children. These were all freshly bereaved people, no more than 2–3 months past the death of their loved ones; the illness and dying experiences were still pretty acute in their minds.

We discussed our plans with the hospital institutional review board, which agreed with our view that the focus groups were being convened as an educational activity, similar to what our health system marketing department does when it assesses patient satisfaction. We used a consent form, however, which told the participants what they would be asked about and that their responses would be kept anonymous, would not be attributed to them without their specific permission and would be used to educate staff and to deliver better care to other patients and families. We developed a semistructured set of questions, which moved from fairly open-ended questions asking them to tell us whatever *they* thought was important, to more specific questions about those issues *we* thought were important. For example, we began by asking, "How did it go? What was important to you?" Then we asked such questions as, "How was your loved one's pain managed? Was the staff helpful and supportive?"

WHAT WE LEARNED FROM THE FOCUS GROUPS

We tape recorded the sessions and then our core Decisions group read the transcripts and analyzed the data to identify the main themes. Through a process of consensus, we culled it down into nine major themes, described here in no particular order:

- **Living with a life-threatening illness is a dynamic, continually evolving experience for the patient and family.**
  The dynamic, evolving aspect of the experience is best summarized by the woman who said, "I never believed my husband was really going to die until the mortuary came to take his body away." The focus group participants really emphasized that, even though they were living with what seemed to be a certainty, it just didn't feel real until it became obvious.

- **The unit of care is the patient *and* family, not just the patient.**
  The family caregivers really emphasized this point. They had many complaints about how hard it was to feel that they were a part of what was going on. They often felt that all the activity and decision making were directed at their loved ones without appropriate recognition of their role.

- **Personalized communication and obtaining information were key issues to family caregivers.**
  Two levels of communication were mentioned: One was the communication and sharing of information between the patient/family and the physician. If you

ask patients and families the question, "How do you feel about the care you received?" they tend to say, "It was wonderful. Everybody was wonderful." But when you ask, "Tell me exactly how did the communication go when you would be in the doctor's office?" they would say, "The doctor was a wonderful human being, but he only spent 10 minutes with us and never answered our questions," and so forth. Families wanted personalized communication: "What will happen to us?" They wanted information that was honest and provided with empathy; they wanted a dialogue. And often, none of those things happened.

Also, families told us, "Each of us has a particular style. Professional caregivers need to recognize our style and assist us in however we do things." So, they emphasized that we, as caregivers, need to recognize how to support that particular family, rather than acting as if there were just one way to do things.

- **In making decisions, most family caregivers and patients followed what the doctors told them to do.**

I asked the focus groups, "How did you make the decisions you made?" In our group, which was pretty much a white middle-class group, almost without exception the answer was that they did what the doctor told them to do. The vast majority, particularly people over the age of 70, didn't quite understand what I meant when I asked, "How did you make decisions?" They looked at me as if to say, "What do you mean? The doctor told us what to do, and we did it, and that's how we do it." In the younger group, there was a lot more dissonance. A small number of people said, "You know, I went in and told the doctor that I've just been on the Internet and asked if my wife should be considered for a stem-cell transplant. In fact, she'd still be alive today, if he had listened to me, but he had started her on standard chemo and she wasn't eligible." They complained, but still did what the doctor told them to do. Then, another group of people said, "I can't believe I did what the doctor told us to do. If I knew then what I know now, I would never have done it, and I didn't like it, and everything we went through was awful, but I did it anyway."

So although there's variation, in the end, people just do what doctors tell them to do, even though the doctors don't realize necessarily that that's what's happening. Physicians think they're giving options, but they're not. It became clear in the focus groups that how information is exchanged and how that exchange leads to decision making was a very complex, hard topic, with many aspects that went beyond just the medical care.

- **Caregiving is an awesome responsibility, but it has enormous rewards.**

The family survivors talked about the incredible demands placed on them by being at home, taking care of this sick person, the fatigue and depression, and just the overwhelming nature of it on one level, and then the incredible rewards on the other level. Their descriptions brought to life the vicissitudes of their situations.

- **Personalized professional caring with empathy was extremely supportive to the patient and family.**

When we asked, "What were the best experiences that you had?" almost universally, the family caregivers said, "Hospice was the best experience we had during a very bad time." Why? "Because it was a personalized experience—people came into our homes, understood our values, and helped us based on our own terms." Everybody thought that was marvelous.

However, responses broke into two groups, the vast majority that had had hospice care and the minority that had not. About two thirds of the group that had received hospice care said, "We wished it would have happened sooner than the last ten days of life." Only five percent of those who had had hospice care had it for longer than that. The other group said, "No one ever offered us hospice."

I asked those people who said they wished hospice care had happened sooner, "Did anybody offer it to you sooner?" Almost two thirds of them said, "Yes. But we weren't ready." It was some kind of defeat or admission of mortality that they weren't yet ready to make. One third of the group said, "No one ever offered it to us, but if they had, we never would have gone through all the horror and hell we went through the last few weeks of my loved one's life, because it was so awful." Now, whether or not it was really offered, who knows? They didn't hear the offer in any case. So, then I said, "Well, how did you get into hospice, then?" And, all of them said, "Well, the doctor or someone in the health care team came up to us and they didn't say, 'Would you like hospice?' They said, 'You need hospice. It's time. You need it now.'"

They made it clear that it wasn't an autonomous choice; it was the strong recommendation from the health care team "knowing you, this is in your best interest" that led them to do it. That really opened my eyes. As a hospice medical director, I had always thought that if we just kept educating the physicians, we would get more people into hospice care. That may still be true, but it hasn't seemed to work that way yet. What the family caregivers really opened up for me is that the meanings ascribed, the way we communicate, and how decisions are made are much more complex and difficult than I had previously understood. I also realized that professional caregivers can be a guide to let people know where they're going and give them some options on how to get there.

The theme of personalized caregiving did not refer to hospice care alone. Rather, it's the idea that care that is really personalized to the needs of the patient/family is remembered as the best experience. For example, one family sneaked the dying patient's dog into the cancer ward and the man died a few hours later with the dog beside him on the bed. People remember that. They also strongly remember interactions with the nursing staff in general, the inpatient/outpatient nursing staff, and the social work and counseling staff as positive events, because these interactions were personalized to the needs of the patient and the family.

• **Grief, loss, and bereavement begin as soon as the patient and family learn that they are facing a life-threatening illness and, for the family, these emotions last beyond the patient's death. Therefore, support—particularly bereavement support—is very important.**

A secondary message was that understanding what the past issues of loss have been for the survivors or the patients is very important. Their past issues of loss have a big impact on how this experience goes for them.

- **Coping mechanisms—what professional caregivers can do to help support people, as well as what the patient and family can do themselves to help them get through the experience—are important.**

Family members mentioned a variety of things professional caregivers can do to help them cope, ranging from the physician making a home visit to the interaction with the mortician. Other means of coping that were mentioned include reading, faith, humor, art, being with family and friends, and community resources.

- **Legal and insurance issues were confusing and difficult.**

Everybody talked about how confusing and difficult the legal and financial aspects of care were. We were impressed with how creative people were in dealing with some significant financial issues. With regard to legal issues, advance directives were important for many of the people in our focus groups, but almost all of them said that the doctor didn't bring the subject up; rather, they took it to the doctor. They told the doctor, "We've been thinking about advance directives and here's what we think." But, in no case did the doctor initiate the discussion.

Based on those nine themes, we began to think about how we could use what the family caregivers had told us to teach other patients and families who are at the beginning, rather than the end, of the experience.

KSH: *How did you develop the workbook for patients and families?*

SF: In the focus groups, we were hearing from people at the end of a long and complex journey. We thought the information we had gained from the focus groups would be useful but, in thinking about giving it to patients and families, we needed to consider their emotional development and the context in which they were living their lives. If you've just learned that you have a life-threatening illness, that is different from having gone through a series of treatments, and you're in the group of people who really aren't getting a lot better, which, in turn, is different from being at the end of the road, down to the last few days or weeks where it's clear that you're not going to survive this illness and your life is going to be foreshortened considerably. So, we began to think, "We'll need to have different instruments or vehicles to help people at different stages." One way to do that would be to have a notebook where you could add pages.

We also wanted to provide information to people in a way that would be meaningful, given where they were in the disease trajectory. It became clear that when they receive cancer diagnoses, patients and families are just pretty much overwhelmed. They're not thinking, "Well, I need to do A, B, and C." They're thinking, "Oh, my God . . . how am I going to get from moment A to moment B?" So we wanted to break the information down into themes and then use the themes in an experiential kind of exercise to help the patient/family discover whatever it is that might be helpful to them. Then, we (the professional care providers) can look at what they've written and discover something about the patient and family.

By this time, we had expanded our initial core group to include representatives from other parts of the organization, which provided opportunities for the cross-fertilization of ideas. We had some pediatric staff who told us that they provide a book, which includes a list of the patient's medications, appointments, and treatment recommendations, to the families of chronically ill or disabled children. They said this book has become a bible to the families of these pediatric patients. That cross-fertilization led us to the idea of a workbook that also would serve as a diary. It would contain exercises designed to elicit statements about who the patient and family are, who should be included in communication and decision making about the patient's medical care, and their treatment goals. After the patients and families finished their work in the notebooks by completing the exercises, we could present distillations to the medical professionals who are providing care to those patients and families, so they would know more about what these patients and families believe.

KSH: *What is the content of the workbook?*

SF: As a subcommittee of the larger task force, we first drafted the workbook to reflect the themes that we identified from what the focus groups had told us. Then, we tested it by giving it first to a few of the people in the focus groups and then to a few people who were in various stages of being ill. Based on the feedback we received, we realized that what patients and families needed was a practical guide.

So the workbook is now being completed by a group of talented writers and educators who are experienced in producing materials for patients and families. These writers simplified and rearranged the material in the workbook so that it would be emotionally appropriate for people who have just learned they have life-threatening illnesses. The material is presented in nonlinear fashion. I describe it in the introduction as follows, "This is filled with information from people who have already been down the path you're going, but everyone is different, and information that's important really varies from person to person and moment to moment. We have designed this workbook so you can go to any page, anywhere, at any time, and do what's important to you right now. All the information in the workbook may eventually be important to you."

The workbook is entitled *Living with a Serious Illness*. It contains an introduction that provides the background and it has a series of sections. The first section, Information and Communication, includes "Getting the Information You Need," "Talking with Your Doctor," and "Let's Talk About Me." Decisions, the second section, includes "Decision Making," "Family and Friends," and "Allowing Help." Resources (health care, community, and financial) is the third section. The Journal, the fourth section, includes a medical journal and a personal journal. One of the major goals of the workbook is to elicit a brief personal statement from the patient about who he or she is, which then can guide the medical staff and caregivers who may have never met the patient, toward understanding a little more about the person as opposed to his or her disease.

In the section on Decisions, under "Family and Friends," we ask, "How are you going to make decisions and who do you want to be involved in that?" Part of that work is to say who your family is, who in that family is going to be an integral, intimate part of supporting you in this experience, and what role do you want that person to play? In that section of the workbook, the patient can say, "This is my disease, and I'm going to make all the decisions, and no one else. I don't want you to talk to anybody." Or, one can say, "I've got a wife, a son, and a daughter, and they're very important. I want them intimately involved in any decisions we make. I want their input, and I want you to talk to them and make sure that they're involved." The patients can say whatever they want, but the workbook raises those issues and allows people to go through a process of first defining, "Who is my family? Who do I want to be involved in this? How do I want them to be involved in this?" Then, "Now that I've decided that, here's a place to summarize what I would like my professional caregivers to know about how my family should be involved in decision making." That's the page that we get, which we would share with our professional caregivers so that they can personalize how they interact with the patient and family.

In the Decisions section, we really emphasize goals. Is your goal to live to the last possible second? Or is your goal to live as long as you can until the burdens become too great? What do you define as burdens? Is your goal to be at home and with your family and to be comfortable and to avoid any medical treatment unless it has a meaningful outcome? It's really to help patients and families understand and express their goals clearly, so that when they go back to the physicians, the physicians can understand what this means to the patients and families.

KSH: *Is there going to be an opportunity for people to change their minds about what's important to them, depending on where they are in the trajectory?*

SF: Absolutely. That's inherent in the conception of the workbook and in the training. Remember, one of the themes from the focus groups was that living with a life-threatening condition is a constantly evolving situation. Therefore, in the training for staff we will stress that health care professionals should always say to patients and families, "You have put down here that this is your goal. Is it still your goal? Is there anything that's changed?"

KSH: *How will the workbook be used in the clinical setting?*

SF: We would like the information provided by the patients through their notebooks to be crosspollinated across their providers, but this has not yet been implemented. Based on the model provided by the pediatric notebook that families carry with them, we are planning to have our adult patients and families carry with them a simple binder or a single page that contains a distillation of whatever they've written in the workbook about themselves and their goals of care. This will be presented in a form that is concise, easy to read, and well-organized so that the health care provider can look at it in 5 minutes and know an enormous amount of information about how this family works and what it wants. When the patient and family meet a new health care professional for the first time, they'll say, "Before you talk to me, I want you to read this stuff and then we can have a conversation."

One item they would carry would be their personal statements. The workbook asks the patient to respond to the question, "If someone providing you with medical care was meeting you for the first time, what would you want them to know about you and your family?" We give them a variety of ways of expressing that: something written, a poem, a piece of art, something that is a work in progress. People can change it, add to it, or subtract from it as they progress through their illness experiences. Another thing they would carry would be lists of the medications they're taking, based on what they actually take and how often as opposed to what we think they take—in other words, something that just says: "Here's your medications. How are you taking them?" The third thing that we would want—and again, that would always be a work in progress—would be a goal statement: Here's what I'm trying to accomplish with my treatment. For example, "I'm out here to live. I want to be cured. That's my goal." Or, "I want to live as long as I can but, if these things happen, then I might not want to live. Let's talk about it again." There might be other kinds of goals, such as, "I want my family, my wife, and my children to be a part of this." Whatever that patient feels is important as a goal would be presented on one sheet, very condensed, which that patient would carry with him or her and make sure, at the beginning of every encounter, that the health care provider takes a very short amount of time to review.

KSH: *Where are you now in the process of developing and implementing the workbook?*

SF: The workbook has great potential, but if we don't implement it softly and well, it can fail incredibly easily and be one more piece of paper that people get that sits on a shelf somewhere doing nothing.

Our goal is to create something that can be used across the system in which these patients are receiving care. We have focused first on people with cancer diagnoses and the parts of the system in which they receive care—for example, the outpatient cancer clinic, the inpatient unit, the radiation therapy unit, and the home health and hospice programs. Later, we may adapt the workbook to be used by people with other life-threatening diagnoses.

The goal is for people to be able to use this workbook on their own, so that they don't have to have someone come in to train or facilitate it. So, the next step is to give the workbook to ten patients and families who are at the beginning of their journeys with life-threatening cancers and see what they think of the workbook. We will field test it, get feedback in a focus group from the people who used the workbook, and then remodel it. We will continue that process until we feel that we have a good product.

After we have a final product, we will determine what we need to do to alter how we deliver medical care to support a process that grounds medical decision making in the values and goals of the patients and families as opposed to those of the medical providers and the systems of care we now have. We need to think about how this workbook can fit into our system and how to ensure that health care providers actually pay attention to it. And we need to train our staff to use it.

Then, the next step is to conduct a training for our whole staff—nurses, radio-therapy techs, support staff, and physicians—about how we're going to use this workbook in our system. It's going to take considerable flexibility and creativity to figure out how this training will work because the physicians have to buy in.

KSH: *What barriers do you perceive now to successful implementation of the workbook?*

SF: Number one is physician buy-in and participation. That is potentially an enormous barrier to which we need to be very sensitive. It's not insurmountable, but we really need to understand that physicians have their own needs and issues, and we want to make sure that this workbook isn't used as a bludgeon to say, "You're not sensitive people; you need to listen to this." It should, instead, become a tool for them to hear and understand patient/family concerns and really lift a burden off physicians and make it easier for them.

In general, physicians have great difficulty in giving patients the cue that it's time to stop treatment. But physicians usually have no difficulty hearing the cue from the patients and families. When they say, "You know what? I don't want to do this anymore," generally physicians feel relieved. Through the use of the workbook, we're trying to make it easy for the patients to give physicians the cues that they're ready for whatever they're ready for and then make it easier for the physicians to follow those cues.

> *Physician backing is key to the success of this innovation. The physicians have been kept aware of the project, but they have not been integral to the development of the notebook. If we do all this and the physicians still remain insulated, it's not going to work, because after all, they are the major drivers of treatment. In our setting, in general, the oncologists are very busy doing oncology and issues in end-of-life care are not high on their radar screens.*

Physician backing is key to the success of this innovation. The physicians have been kept aware of the project, but they have not been integral to the development of the notebook. If we do all this and the physicians still remain insulated, it's not going to work, because after all, they are the major drivers of treatment. In our setting, in general, the oncologists are very busy doing oncology and issues in end-of-life care are not high on their radar screens.

So, it's really important how we do this. We're already starting to sit down with physicians and say, "Here's where we're at. What are your issues and problems?" and then, come back with, "We have a product that can help you with your problems." We've already begun these discussions with physicians, starting with the medical director, who was quite responsive to considering the ways in which the patient workbook might help. And one oncologist is a real champion and very supportive of the project.

The other barrier is finding the time to keep moving forward on the project, which is an add-on to everybody's daily life. You still have to do everything you normally do. So, maintaining the energy and focus to get it done in the busy hustle-and-bustle of an ever-changing and demanding world of medical delivery is a challenge for everybody.

Another barrier is that, as this becomes known and its positive potential becomes clear, then everybody says, "This is a great idea! We'd like to do this in the open-heart surgery, and we would like to do this in the neonatal intensive care unit, and we would like to do this in wherever." And so we need to be able to say, "Whoa! That's great, but implementation of something like this is complex, so we're just going to focus on cancer patients to start with, and we're going to wait until we really know what we're doing there, and have been successful, before we broaden it to other constituencies in the organization." I think it's important to remain really focused on doing a small well-done project rather than trying to do too much.

I don't know if it's a barrier, but in preparation for this project and others spawned by the Decisions Task Force, we went to our administration and said, "We're going to be doing these projects and we want your support." We went to the chief operating officer, who asked some very astute questions. We got her agreement that, if we could show that this thing was doing something positive for the organization and for the patients, then she would back us up. In other words, if a physician said, "You know, I don't want to do this," and we've demonstrated what a great benefit it is, then she would come down and say, "I'm sorry you don't want to do this, but you need to do this."

KSH: *How is the project being funded?*

SF: This is mainly being funded through small grant money, with a small amount through the hospital administration. I think that's been a barrier. If we had had appropriate resources, the workbook would already have happened. Once we have the final workbook to go forward with, then we'll go for big grants to produce it and to do the initial training of health care providers to use it.

KSH: *How will you measure the success of this project?*

SF: We are now thinking about what might be appropriate measures of success. I think there should be some indicators other than patient and provider satisfaction, some endpoints that we would hope to see. We need to think of something that's not very complex and is pretty measurable.

Clearly, however, we're going to measure satisfaction, which, in our organization, is measured by the marketing department in a sophisticated way. One of the reasons our pain management program was so well supported by the hospital administration was because the marketing department found that if patients were extremely satisfied that their pain was well-managed, then they were devout supporters of Multicare. That did more than any other argument I had to get the administration's backing for our pain management program.

At any rate, that is certainly something we need to think about as we go into implementation, to see how the workbook will affect outcomes.

KSH: *Will the workbook be helpful to people who aren't very literate or to those from different ethnic backgrounds?*

SF: I think the workbook is capable of being modified for particular groups. It can be simplified for people who aren't literate. It offers the provider, such as the social worker or the nurse, who already have the job of trying to determine the patients' values and coping abilities, a systematic way of understanding what is important to the patient and the family. So, I think you could sit down and train staff to use this approach in a culturally sensitive way, as a set of exercises, with people who are unable to read or write English well. I think that, in different ethnic, and particularly in disadvantaged socioeconomic groups, we would depend more on developing relationships with somebody trusted to be a facilitator of communication with the patients and families. It would be much more verbal or relationship-driven than just handing them a workbook and saying, "Go through it." At least initially, we would want to learn basic information, such as, "How do you want to communicate? Whom do we communicate with in your family? And what are we going to communicate about?"

With a Native American, you could ask, "How do you want to talk about something if you're really sick?" That person might say, "We don't really talk about being really sick." Then you would say, "Well, when you're sick, whom do you want me to talk to? Do you want me to talk to you or other people in your family, or whom else?" Certainly, just asking the questions about who the patient is, who the family is, who the patient wants to be involved in decision making, and how that patient wants health care providers to communicate with her or her and the family about the patient's illness would be very valuable.

What I've learned from all my research really boils down to this: Everybody has a certain process of awareness. Through that awareness, people connect to the world and their experiences. If you, as a health care provider, don't know what their processes of awareness are and how they connect to the world, you're very handicapped in how you're going to work with these patients. The workbook is a way to help any patient or family members identify what shapes their own awareness and any health care providers figure out how they're going to connect to those patients and families.

You want to ask very neutral, open questions that allow people to fill in for you their contexts of awareness and how they connect to them. You could do it in writing, or with a videotape, or audiotape, or anything. The real idea is to accentuate awareness that then allows you to connect to the experience. That's the process that underlies whatever technique or form that we're using. The workbook is merely a vehicle for doing that.

KSH: *What changes, if any, in your medical care delivery system do you think would be needed to support this project?*

SF: Probably the weakest link in medical care is the lack of a systematic or any kind of continuity among provider points. It's just an incredible problem. As Ira Byock, MD, pointed out recently at a conference I attended, "The way medicine is organized is that you get maximum reimbursement for individuals doing their individual treatment of their individual part of an illness, and you get very little reimbursement for any kind of continuity." So, I think that's just an inherent problem in what we do, and one of the positive sides of the recent changes in the delivery and organization of medicine is that now there is a system, which provides an opportunity to improve continuity of care.

I work for a hospital that is providing many services under the same corporate banner. In trying to improve care near the end of life, our first step was to use the system by including on our Decisions Task Force representatives from each part of the system. We've brought together people from radiotherapy, pharmacy, nursing, the oncology inpatient and outpatient units, hospice, and home health care. At least, we have all those players around the table talking about a project that would benefit care in a way that we can all be a part of.

I don't think we're trying to change our system. What we're trying to do is to recognize that we have a system and to develop our project so as to take advantage of what's already there.

REFERENCE

1. Farber S, Anderson W, Braden C, Isenhower P, Lanier K, O'Reiley L. Improving cancer pain management through a system wide commitment. *J Palliative Med* 1998;1(4): 377-385.

International Perspectives

Common Sense

LESLIE J. BLACKHALL, MD, MTS

Assisted Home Hospice
Thousand Oaks, California

I was asked to write an essay about cultural diversity, but as I began to write, I realized that it was really about *common sense*. Common sense is the truth we do not question. When someone makes a statement and then says "that's common sense," that person means that there is no need for any further justification. It is self-evident. I guess one could say that doing research into cultural diversity has made me lose my common sense.

I am a hospice physician and a researcher who has lectured and published widely about the ethical and practical aspects of caring for dying patients. Several years ago my colleagues (Gelya Frank, PhD; Sheila Murphy, PhD; Vicki Michel, JD; and Stan Azen, PhD) and I completed a large project called Ethnicity and Attitudes Toward Care at the End of Life. This study examined attitudes toward a variety of topics related to the care of dying patients (truth telling, patient autonomy, advance care directives, and withholding and withdrawing care) among elderly subjects from four different ethnic groups: Mexican-American, Korean-American, African-American, and white (European-American). In the first part of this study, we interviewed 800 subjects, 200 in each group, using a standardized questionnaire. They answered yes or no, agree or disagree; they picked from multiple choices. In this way, we got a lot of information about our subjects' beliefs and values as well as about their demographic characteristics. We were able to do statistical analyses to see how attitudes differed and if those attitudes differed by ethnic group or if those differences could be attributed to something else, such as socioeconomic status or religion. But, because we recognized that attitudes about something as complex as the dying process cannot necessarily be reduced to multiple-choice questions, we went back the next year to talk to 10 percent of the participants of our original group in an indepth ethnographic format. These interviews, conducted by anthropologists, got something more than answers; the interviews got people's *stories*, their experiences, and the meanings they made of those experiences.

> *When we say that something is common sense, we mean that it is an idea that makes so much sense to us that we have never examined it; perhaps it is the idea that was so ingrained in us from earliest childhood, so reinforced by our culture that we cannot think to question it.*

I initiated this project because I was convinced that we in the bioethics profession were missing something. I was beginning to feel that many of the assumptions underlying attempts to improve care at the end of life were based on the experience of the mostly white middle-class professionals, like myself, who did bioethics. We assumed, for example, that people are concerned with getting too much care at the end of life, and desire protection from overburdensome care, perhaps in the form of advance care directives. Working at the Los Angeles County Hospital, it seemed unlikely that this was the major concern of the poor, mainly Latino patients for whom I cared.

The results of this study surpassed my expectations, but certain types of criticism stymied me. Were we just stereotyping? How could statistical information about the beliefs of a whole group help us with our encounters with individual patients? My greatest fear about our study was that the results would be reduced to a 4×6 inch index card in a medical student's pocket: Korean people, don't tell; Mexican-American, don't tell; White and African-American, tell. Then again, after lectures people frequently came up complaining that we had not mentioned the group they were most concerned with: Armenians, H'mong people, and Russian Jews. Was the point of this work to study, in detail, the beliefs of every group in the United States? Was this possible, or even desirable?

Despite these concerns, I still knew that we and others in the field were doing something important, that if we didn't listen to these voices we would be missing something crucial. Then, one day, while standing in my office reading a transcript, I had an epiphany. I was puzzling over a problem with the way our Korean-American subjects had answered some of the questions in our survey. The vast majority of them, close to 80 percent, agreed with statements such as: "You should always keep a patient on life support, even if it appears hopeless, because there is always a chance of a miracle." (By contrast, very few white subjects will agree with this statement.) On the other hand, very few of the Korean elderly people we interviewed (only approximately 5 percent) wished personally to be put on life support at the end of their lives. What could this contradiction mean? No matter how I looked at it, I could not make sense of these results. So, we asked our anthropologists, as part of their interviews, to bring this issue up with the Korean subjects to whom they talked. The first of these interviews, transcribed and translated, were now coming in. In the transcript I was holding, a patient we have called Mrs. Kim explained her views, which I paraphrase here. "I, myself, would not want to be kept alive by life support," she said. "But I would be the dying patient, so it wouldn't be my choice. My children would decide, and they would have to keep me alive even one more day; that is the right behavior for children." She went on to tell us that, if people heard that a child had decided to do anything else for a parent, this would be regarded as "unfilial." Similarly, although she acknowledged that, in the abstract, it might be good to let a patient die sooner, with less pain, she would always ask the doctors to keep her aging parents or sick child alive even one more day.[1][†]

[†]For a longer and more thorough discussion of this case, see Reference 1 at the end of this chapter.

Reading this, I suddenly realized that what seemed like a contradiction to me was only a contradiction because I was viewing the issue through the lens of patient autonomy. It seemed self-evident to me that the patient's wishes were of paramount importance in making a decision about life support. But, to Mrs. Kim, her wishes were not the crucial factor. The relevant ethical principle was "*hyodo*," filial piety. In the case of her illness, it would be the duty of her children to care for her and the appropriate way for them to show their caring would be to keep her alive, even one more day. Looking at these seemingly conflicting answers to our questionnaire through the lens of *hyodo*, the conflict dissolves. These elderly Korean-Americans do not want to be kept alive on life support *and* they think it is the right thing that people be kept on life support. Should their family members do any less for them, it would show a lack of caring that would shame the family, and perhaps, cause them to feel unloved.

> *Reading this, I suddenly realized that what seemed like a contradiction to me was only a contradiction because I was viewing the issue through the lens of patient autonomy.*

Mostly, I have not changed my own beliefs about how I would like to be cared for at the end of my life. But I have stopped believing that the good death I envision for myself is a death that would seem good to someone else. I have come to distrust the idea of "common sense." When we say that something is common sense, we mean that it is an idea that makes so much sense to us that we have never examined it; perhaps it is the idea that was so ingrained in us from earliest childhood, so reinforced by our culture that we cannot think to question it. Almost all of our subjects, whatever ethnic group they are from, think dying people know they are dying. To the African-American and European-American subject, it is "common sense," therefore, that one can tell them that they are dying. Why hide the truth being that they already know it? But to our Korean-American and Mexican-American subjects, it is "common sense" that, for this very reason, one does not need to tell them. Why cause them more pain?

Common sense is the lens through which I see the world, the lens I have worn so long that I have forgotten that it *is* a lens. Doing this study allowed me to see that I do wear a lens, a straight-white-girl-from-Schenectady lens. And the study allowed me, for a few moments here and there, to take off my lens and try on someone else's. The subjects in this study enlarged my vision, and for that, I will be forever grateful.

REFERENCE

1. Frank G, Blackhall L, Michel V, Murphy S, Azen S, Park K. A discourse of relationships in bioethics: Patient autonomy and end of life decision making among elderly Korean Americans. *Med Anthropol Q* 1998;12(4):403–423.

Excerpted from the Online Discussion,
Innovations in End-of-Life Care
Volume 1, Number 2, April 2, 1999

On Cultural Diversity and "Common Sense":
A Case Example in Hospice Care

Leslie J. Blackhall, MD, MTS
Assisted Home Hospice
Thousand Oaks, California

I received a referral for a patient from El Salvador who had a recurrence of esophageal cancer. He was in excruciating pain and had waited all day in the County Hospital emergency room only to be sent home with Tylenol with codeine, which, needless to say did nothing for him and he was curled up in a fetal position. My nurse was dispatched out there and we got him started on something more effective and he was feeling much better—up and about and eating little bits of food. He and his family were incredibly grateful for the personal attention and the symptom control. The only problem was, we couldn't seem to get him to sign the papers that would get him officially into hospice care.

As soon as I heard the story I knew what must be up. The family would talk to the nurse in English and thank her effusively, but when it came to have them translate the consent forms to the patient (he spoke no English and this nurse spoke little Spanish), they would get vague and defer to another time. So, I called to tell them I was coming out and the panicked daughter told me, please not to tell him that he had less than 6 months to live (this is, of course, on the hospice consent forms), because I would kill him. He did know his cancer had recurred and had told his family previously that he never wanted to do chemotherapy again. When I got to the house, I found the whole family there. The family members repeated what the daughter had said. So I asked the patient if he was the kind of guy who wanted to make all his decisions himself and know everything about his illness or did he prefer to leave that to his family. He readily agreed that his family should handle things and he trusted them. I told him I would always be willing to answer any questions about his care. He told me he had none. Then the son told him to sign the papers (without translations), and he did.

We continued to care for him for several months and I visited him from time to time. I would always ask if he had questions, and he occasionally did, but they were of this sort: "Can I eat ice cream?" and "Is it okay to take additional pain medicine at night?"

I learned so much from this case. One thing I learned was about communication. This gentleman, in my opinion, knew exactly what was going on with him. At one point he told his children, who told me, that he wanted to die in El Salvador. So, when he was deteriorating but still strong enough to get on a plane, we sent him home. Communication was occurring. The number of his family members who were present all the time, the care they took with him—all this must have been telling him that he was dying. In this context, the family's refusal to discuss his prognosis openly was also a communication, a message to him about how much the family members cared. They cared enough to protect him from news that could only make him unhappy and hasten his demise. When I told him that it was time to go to El Salvador, I too, was communicating, even though we never overtly discussed why this was so.

To help this man properly did require a lot of staff education because there is the hospice model of open communication and truthfulness being the key to care. In general, I think that hospice patients tend to be less culturally diverse than the general population because of the perception that hospice care takes away hope. I am working hard in our community to dispel this perception, and I think it will require working closely with members of the diverse communities to be able to serve them in the way they prefer to be cared for, rather than trying to impose our model of a good death.

Cancer Disclosure and Family Involvement with Japanese Patients in the United States

MICHAEL D. FETTERS, MD, MPH, MA

Japanese Family Health Program
Ann Arbor, Michigan

Michael D. Fetters, MD, MPH, MA, is a family physician and director of the Japanese Family Health Program in Ann Arbor, Michigan, where he cares for many Japanese expatriates. Dr. Fetters lived in Japan for almost 3 years. As a Fulbright scholar there, he conducted research on physician disclosure of cancer diagnoses to patients and families. This experience, and his fluency in Japanese, have provided him with a particular expertise and a lens for identifying dilemmas that can arise when caring for Japanese patients in the United States. In the following piece, adapted from an interview conducted by Anna L. Romer, he first describes the knowledge that his research on family decision making and cancer disclosure in Japan offered him as a practicing physician. Then he provides a case example that illuminates the complexity that such knowledge adds when the two relevant cultural, linguistic, and legal systems lead to contradictory, or at least distinct, paths of action.

I first went to Japan as a teenager through the American Field Service, an international exchange program, and I have been there many times since. As a Fulbright scholar, I conducted research on end-of-life decision making there. Prior to conducting this research, I was familiar with the idea that it was common not to disclose a cancer diagnosis in Japan. However, when I got to Japan, I observed that the family took on what seemed to be a very different role in decision making from that in the United States. This different ethic regarding cancer disclosure was like a light through a cracked door, that led me to a new place. It was an invitation to reexamine family decision making and how families are much more the unit of care in practice in the Japanese setting than in the American setting.

Here in Ann Arbor, Michigan, I'm a family physician, involved in the care of patients across the life span, from babies to geriatric patients. While end-of-life care is a small percentage of my practice, I am involved in the care of dying patients. A large number of my patients are Japanese: anywhere from 70 to 80 percent most clinic days, and some days as much as 100 percent, because I am one of the few physicians in the area who speaks Japanese. We have a large Japanese population because of the automotive industry and because of research and other academic opportunities at the University of Michigan, Ann Arbor.

One of the very difficult things in making cross-cultural comparisons is that there is always the risk of stereotyping. There is enormous heterogeneity in the roles that families assume when they are caring for a loved one or making health decisions. That is true in this country and it is also true in Japan. One of the things that medical anthropology has taught us to do is to really look at the details and the rich diversity that exists within any one culture. Therefore, I am a bit hesitant to say, "This is the way it is in Japan and this is the way it is in the United States." Nevertheless, one can still step back and say there are some very different patterns that emerge regarding the roles that families tend to play in the United States and the roles that families tend to play in Japan. The other thing, obviously, about culture is that it is dynamic, and there are lots of changes occurring in Japan at this time, which will affect doctor–patient communication.

DIFFERENT APPROACHES TO PATIENTS FROM DIFFERENT CULTURAL BACKGROUNDS

I did not realize I was doing anything differently in terms of my approach to American patients and Japanese patients until I had medical students with me, who asked me questions about why I was taking a particular course of action. At one level, what underlies my approach is the same for all patients, in the sense that I am really trying to understand what the patient's motivations for health care are, what his or her own concerns are, what sorts of explanatory models the patient is using, and what his or her own view is about what is causing the illness. Then I try to figure out how I can integrate the care that I provide to that patient with his or her own explanatory model. So, I really try to take that approach with everyone.

At the same time, I do know quite a bit about Japanese culture, and that puts me at a different starting point when I interact with Japanese patients. I think that understanding a lot about a particular patient population can give you a better starting point for finding out where it is that patients stand on particular issues and where they want to go. However, that knowledge can also complicate things when it is used in a crosscultural setting.

AMBIGUOUS DISCLOSURE

Ambiguous disclosure is a concept that comes out of research that Akira Akabayashi, Todd S. Elwyn, and I have done on cancer disclosure.[1] We documented one pattern of how Japanese physicians interact with patients. What it boils down to is that it is very easy in Japanese to give a vague sense of what is going on. Ambiguity is a standard part of the language; in everyday life, conversation is less direct. If conversation is customarily vague, one does not feel as though someone is intentionally trying to deceive one.

Around the issue of cancer disclosure, for example, it is natural to speak rather vaguely about what sorts of things have been found, regarding the physical examination or laboratory work-up using blood tests or the sorts of findings present on X-rays. Ambiguous disclosure, we argue, really becomes an invitation to the patient to determine how much he or she really wants to know about a particular topic. In this sense, ambiguous disclosure allows the listener a choice about how to proceed. The patient can then, in theory, take control and say, "This is something that doesn't make sense to me. You're not painting a completely clear picture of what's going on here. Give me some more details on that." However, what is complicated is that the patient may worry about breaking social norms if he or she inquires too directly in response to ambiguous disclosure. Again, this depends on the circumstance and the approach that a particular physician takes.

SOCIOLINGUISTICS AND CULTURAL KNOWLEDGE

Clearly, another important difference between interactions taking place in English and those in Japanese, whether here or in Japan, has to do with the Japanese language, in which there are hierarchical structures embedded in the language itself. There is a variety of terms to use for expressing the "self"; there is also a variety of terms used for expressing the pronoun "you." The selection of specific terms may humble the speaker or elevate the person being addressed.

These linguistic structures provide important cues that influence where the discussion can or should go. Furthermore, there are honorifics that make a discussion either more formal or less formal. And there are different verbs that one can use, which again, would reflect hierarchical differences. So it gets tricky, especially for someone who is grounded in a different culture, even if that person is "fluent" in Japanese. Understanding the meaning of a conversation on a delicate subject becomes quite dependent on sociolinguistic and cultural knowledge as well as on the assumptions of each speaker. On the one hand, physicians could try speaking at a very familiar level, but patients might then take that to mean, "This is an informal doctor who isn't a good doctor just because he or she is not very doctor-ish." There are many judgment calls about how to address others.

CULTURAL HETEROGENEITY: PATIENTS DIFFER IN HOW MUCH THEY WANT TO KNOW

As I was building my practice of Japanese patients, I was well-versed in issues of ethics and respect for patient autonomy, and I had a personal theory that the reason that patients were not exercising autonomy was because they just had not been given the opportunity in Japan. I soon learned that that was true for some people, but *only* for some people. I have actually been amazed by the number of questions that many of my Japanese patients have about their health. Sometimes, they have even more than I would expect from my English-speaking patients. This experience is very interesting because it was quite common for me to hear Japanese physicians say that patients really do not have any questions, "end of story." In contrast, I have found that patients are frequently very inquisitive. And yet, there is a lot of heterogeneity. Some of my Japanese patients do sound like what Japanese physicians would predict—basically these patients want to follow my advice. When I offer them several treatment options, "Well, we could do this or that," then these patients will come back and say, "Well, which do you think I should do?" Others really want to know everything.

DUAL IDENTITY OFFERS MORE DEGREES OF FREEDOM

The first thing I bring to the interaction is that I am not Japanese, so my patients are allowed to change the rules a bit. The boundaries, all of a sudden, are no longer clear. There is an expectation that I am a Japanese-speaking doctor, who is the director of the Japanese Family Health Program at a clinic where the nurse is Japanese, the receptionist is Japanese, and the other doctor is Japanese. So there is a relatively high expectation that this clinic is Japanese-centered. But, at the same time, I am not Japanese, so the boundaries are ambiguous; one has to explore a bit, I guess, and say, "Where do we draw the lines?" Patients, too, can explore how much they want to participate or how much they are encouraged to participate in decisions about their health care.

CLINICAL TOOL TO ELICIT PREFERENCES:
ADVANCE DIRECTIVE FOR DISCLOSURE

Because of the issue of nondisclosure of cancer diagnoses in Japan, when working with Japanese patients who appeared to be seriously ill, I began using an "advance directive for disclosure." Since I started this practice, others such as Atsushi Asai, for example, have published written versions.[2] I think it says something about the validity of this concept of an advance directive for cancer disclosure that it has cropped up in several places.

This document basically asks the patient for his or her preferred level of participation in decision making. Actually, the document has evolved even since I started using it. Now, I try to find out both to what degree a patient wants to participate in decision making, and how much information the patient wants to know. There is research coming out suggesting that physicians in the United States overestimate the degree to which patients want to participate in decisions, whereas they underestimate the amount of information that patients want to know about their conditions. Working on that assumption, I am raising the same questions with all of my patients, not only my Japanese patients. I want to get both a sense of how much patients want to participate in decisions and how much information they actually want to know.

My original document is in Japanese, in the form of a questionnaire because it was originally a research questionnaire. The conclusion that I have come to is that the written form is much less important than the opportunity that the questions create for a dialogue with the patient. The document allows for an opportunity to explore, "Where is this person coming from? In what direction does he or she want to go?" Now I usually use an oral advance directive for disclosure with patients.

CASE EXAMPLE: A JAPANESE MAN WHO PRESENTS AS GRAVELY ILL AT A JAPANESE CLINIC IN THE UNITED STATES, ACCOMPANIED BY HIS WIFE—WHICH CULTURE'S RULES SHOULD BE FOLLOWED?

EDITORS' NOTE: The indented text tells the story of what happened. The full-page text describes Dr. Fetters' internal dialogue as he balanced different expectations and ethical principles in this interaction with a Japanese patient and his wife. Dr. Fetters presented this case at the American Society of Bioethics and Humanities meeting.[3]

> A middle-aged Japanese man came into my office with his wife complaining of a lump in his stomach. His skin was yellow and he was losing weight. Within the first 30 seconds of the interview, it was clear that he had a very serious problem. Any clinician would look at this person and say, "There's something very serious here; the fact that he is complaining of this hard mass is virtually diagnostic of his having some sort of cancer."

In this case I found myself trying to process all of the information that I had about how different cancer disclosure attitudes are in the United States and Japan. In Japan, there is a tendency to tell breadwinners of the family if they have cancer. Then there is the fact that he's living in the United States, and there are other considerations, too. The question becomes, to what degree am I obligated to follow U.S. expectations and rules versus Japanese expectations for disclosure? And what exactly would those be, in this situation?

I thought I was really prepared for the time when a cancer patient would walk through my door because of all the research I'd done in Japan, especially if the patient were Japanese. Yet, all of a sudden, when the rubber hit the road, I realized again how difficult it all is, despite all the scholarly work I had done. Luckily, the physical examination can be a time-generating opportunity to think.

> I proceeded to ask him his preferred level of involvement in things, and he quickly said, "Well, I want you to tell me everything."

Now this is a helpful question, but it alone does not make the doctor's job easier. When a patient says, "Tell me everything," how much does that really mean? How fast? Should one just dump the whole can of worms here? Should the physician use time as an element to warm up the patient to the diagnosis? Remember, I had no previous relationship with this person. His wife was also with him at the time. They both appeared really very concerned. He was obviously very sick, and I was almost certain he had cancer, and probably at a very bad stage of the disease.

What I decided to do represented a compromise. I was more explicit than ambiguous disclosure would require, but perhaps less explicit than the American norm.

> I gave him a differential diagnosis. It could be hepatitis. (He had had a history of a different kind of hepatitis.) It could also possibly be cirrhosis, because he was a fairly liberal user of alcohol. I mentioned in passing at the very end of the interview, that, well, this could also be a cancer. When I said "cancer," his face dropped. His chin almost hit the floor.

When I saw my patient's shock, I became enormously uncomfortable. On the one hand, I felt, "I've really gone too far here. This is the first time that I've met this person." On the other hand, I felt I was deceiving the patient. I think that this is something that clinicians oftentimes are not honest about with themselves. I had intentionally tucked the possibility of his having cancer all the way at the very end, trying to deemphasize it, using that as a tool for trying to acclimate him to the idea that there could be something very serious here. Strictly speaking, I was honest. I did not really know for certain what he had. I was conveying to him that he had something quite serious. But I did not disclose the full range of my thinking. I did not say, "I really think that you have cancer."

With an American patient, I might have been more candid about the fact that I had a strong suspicion that this was cancer. So really, again, this comes down to the question of whether a physician should do things differently with patients from a different cultural and linguistic background or not.

In Japan, physicians will often divulge a cancer diagnosis to family members first and ask the family whether the diagnosis should be shared with the patient. Consulting with families is seen as appropriate. In fact, physicians are expected to take families' preferences into account. My own unpublished research on the use of advance directives for disclosure showed that virtually everyone who said that they would not want to be told themselves about an advanced stage of cancer said that they would want their spouse told. The data that I had collected among this same population (Japanese expatriates visiting a Japanese-centered clinic in the United States) had told me that the more likely it was that a patient coming for cancer laboratory tests actually had a worse stage of malignant disease, the less likely it was that that patient would want to be told that he or she had cancer. In that circumstance, most patients preferred that their spouses be told.

> In light of this research, one of the things I did was to talk with this patient's wife while he was changing his clothes, when it was natural for us to leave the room. I said, "You know, I think there's a pretty good chance this is cancer and, if it is, do you think it's appropriate to tell him?" And she said, "Absolutely not! Don't tell him. You can't tell him; he would never be able to handle it."

Here is a situation in which I tried to put my research findings into practice. I had asked the wife her opinion on disclosure and received an unequivocal response, "Absolutely don't tell him. It'll kill him. He'll get worse." Yet, I am an American physician, practicing in the United States, and the patient has told me to tell him everything.

I reviewed the differential diagnosis and suggested that he needed to be hospitalized so that we could do the usual diagnostic tests and try to figure out what he had. I explained that they would then come back to the office to talk about the results with me. The patient was then admitted to our university medical hospital.

As it happened, I knew the attending physician on the service, as well as the resident. Because of the size of our institution, it is actually unusual for this to happen. It was the best possible circumstance for taking a coordinated approach that would take into account his cultural background. You cannot go against the flow, if you do not know the people on the inpatient team.

> *"In the United States, we tell patients virtually everything about their care—as much information as they want to know, whereas in Japan, that's not always the case. Because I'm familiar with the traditions in Japan, I want to make sure that we're doing things the way you want to have them done." He said, "Well, I want to know everything." He seemed to be very resolute. There was no trepidation in his voice. So then I told him that it was cancer. He replied, "Well, I thought so."*

In this case, I was able to say, "We're not going to dump everything out on him while he's in the hospital. This is a very sensitive and delicate issue, and I think it's probably best for me to handle his test results in the outpatient setting." All the physicians agreed, given the circumstances, that this was the way to go.

He had a computed tomography (CT) scan of the abdomen, and he was having some diarrhea as a complication of the malignancy, so the hospital team did a workup on that. Basically these tests only took about a day, and so the hospital staff prepared to discharge him that evening.

As is often the case in American hospital settings, there was too little doctor–nurse communication about the patient, and the nursing staff apparently had not been involved in the decision to hold off on the disclosure of test results. As a result, the discharge nurse dutifully pulled out her standard institutional form that lists a series of questions to be answered, namely, "What's the patient's name? What are his or her medications? What's the diagnosis? What did the test results show?" Well, she wrote the answers, as she was supposed to, on the form, including, "There's a 12-cm mass in your liver." After getting his discharge instructions, the patient reported that she said, "You are all set, you can go home now." At this point, it was fairly late at night. The patient took the form, walked into the parking lot with his wife, and broke into tears.

This man had two daughters; it was the birthday of, I believe, his older daughter. Here he is in the hospital getting a CT scan to show that he's got cancer, and his daughter was supposed to be having her birthday party. I am not criticizing the nurse here. In fact, one could blame us, the doctors, for not including the nurses in our plan. However, I see it as an indictment of the whole system. The nurse was doing her job: writing down the diagnosis and giving it to the patient. That is informed consent. That is ethics in practice in the United States.

The patient did follow up with me the next day and told me what had happened. Again, he had a very serious, downtrodden look, and his wife looked the same way.

I reviewed what I understood his preferences to be for disclosure. This conversation was all occurring in Japanese, with me saying, "In the United States, we tell patients virtually everything about their care—as much information as they want to know, whereas in Japan, that's not always the case. Because I'm familiar with the traditions in Japan, I want to make sure that we're doing things the way you want to have them done." He said, "Well, I want to know everything." He seemed to be very resolute. There was no trepidation in his voice. So then I told him that it was cancer. He replied, "Well, I thought so."

This experience made clear to me how murky these questions about decision making are. How do you determine what patients want? What do families want? Who decides what, and who is included in decision making? In the end, this patient was able to return home to Japan expeditiously in part because he brought his boss into my office. Including his boss in the decision making was good for his situation. Once in Japan, his disease was treated more aggressively than it would have been in the United States, where palliative care would likely have been the recommended route.

His wife kept up with me after his death and reported that she felt he died sooner than he needed to, because of those aggressive, curative efforts. She was happy for him, though, because he wanted to have treatment because he wanted to have a chance to live. All in all, I would like to think that I created a positive opportunity for his wife to participate in his care. She was consulted in the same way she would have been in Japan. I hope that including elements of both Japanese and American approaches to care gave her and the patient, her husband, some sense of normalcy.

THE TAKE-HOME MESSAGES OF THIS CASE

As this example makes clear, current principles in ethics fall short in their capacity to guide action on the part of a physician who is operating across two quite different cultural worlds. Which culture's rules should hold? There is more to autonomy than just talking directly with the patient. My definition of respect for patient autonomy is robust, and that means taking into account the patient's preferences, and that means including family members and others if the patient wants them to be involved.

> *My definition of respect for patient autonomy is robust, and that means taking into account the patient's preferences, and that means including family members and others if the patient wants them to be involved.*

Without stereotyping, Japanese physicians tend to talk about making decisions based on a variety of elements and not making decisions based strictly on principles. In the United States, physicians often turn to principles of autonomy to buttress their decisions—for example: "Well, it's their right to know" or "The patient has to know; it's the patient's decision."

There is a place for the use of philosophical principles in medical decision making, but there is also a place for narrative ethics and putting the patient in context and really weighing all of the different factors. When we experience difficulties is when these different approaches lead to different conclusions. The assumption is that there is a lot of room under the rubric of "patient autonomy" to respect all the kinds of issues that narrative ethics, feminist ethics, or a crosscultural perspective might make more salient. The problem is that you can come to very different conclusions depending on what approach you take. We really have not developed a mechanism for understanding when one principle or a conclusion drawn from one or another ethical approach ought to outweigh others. That is the real difficulty.

REFERENCES

1. Akabayaski A, Fetters MD, Elwyn TS. Family consent, communication, and advance directives for cancer disclosure: A Japanese case and discussion. *J Med Ethics* 1999;25:296–301
2. Asai A. Should physicians tell patients the truth? *Western J Med* 1995;163:36–39.
3. Fetters MD. Can U.S. medical culture tolerate non-disclosure of the cancer diagnosis? First American Society of Bioethics and Humanities Meeting, November 1998, Houston, Texas.

Selected Bibliography

Part Three

Selected articles by contributors to this part:

Blackhall LJ, Murphy ST, Frank G, Michel V, Azen S. Ethnicity and attitudes toward patient autonomy. *JAMA* 1995;274(10):820–825.

Elwyn TS, Fetters MD, Gorenflo DW, Tsuda T. Cancer disclosure in Japan: Historical comparisons, current practices. *Soc Sci Med* 1998;46:1151–1163.

Farber S, Anderson W, Branmden C, Isenhower P, Lanier K, O'Reilly L. Improving cancer pain management through a system wide commitment. *J Palliative Med* 1998;1(4):377–385.

Farber S, Herman-Bertsch J. Using standardized patients to teach palliative care principles to primary care residents. *J Cancer Ed* 1998;12(3[suppl]):20.

Fetters MD. The family in medical decision making: Japanese perspectives. *J Clin Ethics* 1998;9:132–146.

Frank G, Blackhall L, Michel V, Murphy S, Azen S, Park K. A discourse of relationships in bioethics: Patient autonomy and end of life decision making among elderly Korean Americans. *Med Anthropol Q* 1998;12(4):403–423.

Other selected literature on cultural diversity in end-of-life decision making:

Accommodating religious and cultural diversity: Tier III essays and annotated Bibliography. In: Solomon et al. (Eds). *Decisions Near the End of Life Faculty Guide.* Decisions Near the End of Life National Coordinating Center at Education Development Center, Newton, MA. 1997.

Asai A. Should physicians tell patients the truth? *Western J Med* 1995;163:36–39.

Asai A, Fukuhara S, Lo B. Attitudes of Japanese and Japanese-American physicians towards life-sustaining treatment. *Lancet* 1995;346:356–359.

Asai A, Kishino M, Fukui T, et al. A report from Japan. Choices of Japanese patients in the face of disagreement. *Bioethics* 1998;12:162–172.

Carrese JA, Rhodes LA. Western bioethics on the Navajo reservation. *JAMA* 1995;274(10):826–829.

Dula A. African American suspicion of the healthcare system is justified: What do we do about it? *Cambridge Q Healthcare Ethics* 1994;3:347–357.

Fadiman A. *The Spirit Catches You and You Fall Down: A H'mong Child, her American Doctors, and the Collision of Two Cultures.* New York: Farrar, Straus, and Giroux, 1997.

Gostin LO. Informed consent, cultural sensitivity and respect for persons. *JAMA* 1995;274(10):844–845.

Hall P, et al. Palliative care: How can we meet the needs of our multicultural communities? *J Palliative Care* 1998;14(2):46–49.

Howard K. Managing diversity. *American Medical News* [Chicago], January 25, 1999, pp. 19-20,22.

Klessig J. The effect of values and culture on life-support decisions. *W J Med* 1992;157:316-322.

Kreier R. Crossing the cultural divide. *American Medical News* [Chicago], January 25, 1999, pp. 10-12.

McDonald-Scott P, Machizawa S, Satoh H. Diagnostic disclosure: A tale in two cultures. *Psychological Med* 1992;22:147-157.

Vawter DE, et al. Hospice care for terminally ill H'mong patients: A good cultural fit? *Minnesota Med* 1997;80(11):42-44.

Other selected literature on the role of families:

DuLac JD, Lynn J. Patient preferences in medical decision making: A collaborative approach. *Quality of Life—A Nursing Challenge* 1994;3:9-13.

Goetschius SK. Families and end-of-life care: How do we meet their needs? *J Gerontol Nurs* 1997;23(3):43-49.

Nelson HL, Nelson JL. *The Patient in the Family: An Ethics of Medicine and Families.* New York: Routledge, 1995.

Nelson JL. Taking families seriously. *Hastings Center Report* 1992;22(4):6-12.

Ramirez A, Addington-Hall J, Richards M. ABC of palliative care: The carers. *Br Med J* 1998;316:208-211.

Yates P, Stetz KM. Families' awareness of and response to dying. *Oncol Nurs Forum* 1999;26(1):113-119.

Part Four

Pain Management

Near the End of Life

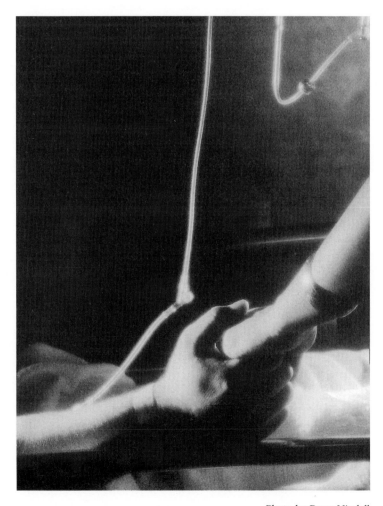

Photo by Doug Mindell

Implementing Pain Management Guidelines

KAREN S. HELLER, PhD

Education Development Center, Inc.
Newton, Massachusetts

The relief of pain and of other symptoms throughout the trajectory of a terminal illness and enhancing the quality of life for patients and their family members remain major challenges. Although it is well known that undertreatment of pain has adverse clinical and quality-of-life effects for patients, pain associated with many life-threatening illnesses, most notably cancer pain, remains seriously undertreated.[1] The reasons for this treatment failure are complex and involve the interrelationship of multiple barriers involving health care professionals, patients, the public, and the health care and legal systems. Among the barriers recently summarized by Foley[2] are: knowledge deficits among clinicians about how to assess and treat cancer pain; widespread fears among clinicians, patients and the public about possible adverse consequences resulting from the prescription of opiates, including concerns about side effects and fears of addiction; legal restrictions on prescribing opiates and clinicians' concerns about legal liability; and, in some countries, lack of access to opiates.[3] Moreover, effective pain management in clinical settings has been hampered by the absence of documented pain assessments and a lack of clear accountability for relieving pain.[4] Until very recently, the relief of pain has been given low priority in health care institutions, with few economic resources committed to treating pain and a lack of policies to support the use of validated pain-measurement tools in clinical practice.[5]

In recent years there has been growing awareness of the need to provide better pain and symptom management, particularly for cancer patients, throughout the course of this disease. Advances in knowledge about the pathophysiology of cancer pain and the availability of validated pain measurement tools now make it possible to provide adequate pain relief to cancer patients.[2] There also has been growing recognition worldwide that many aspects of palliative care are applicable earlier in the course of illness in conjunction with anticancer treatment. As the Institute of Medicine's Committee on Care at the End of Life observed, "it is not enough to emphasize control of symptoms once they are well-established. If identified and impeccably managed earlier in the trajectory of illness, many of the symptom problems that afflict dying patients could be either eliminated or more readily managed."[1] Early aggressive treatment of pain, before it becomes intractable, is now recognized to be extremely important if adequate control is to be achieved.

During the 1980s and early 1990s in the United States, educational efforts to improve pain management was targeted first to nurses and then to physicians, with little initial effect, which led many researchers to conclude that professional education alone was insufficient to change practice.[6] Recent efforts have focused on a combination of professional education and continuous-quality improvement efforts as well as institutionalizing better pain management through such measures as increased documentation of pain assessment and treatment.[7,8] National guidelines on the treatment of cancer pain underscore that pain management is not just the responsibility of individual clinicians; institutions are accountable for having structures and processes in place to ensure that patients have access to appropriate pain management. The American Pain Society,[9] the U.S. Agency for Healthcare Research and Quality (AHRQ) [formerly the U.S. Agency for Health Care Policy and Research (AHCPR)][10] and the Oncology Nursing Society[11] all have recognized the role institutions play in improving pain management and made recommendations directed at institutional structures and processes. The Joint Commission on the Accreditation of Hospitals recently set institutional standards for pain management.[12]

In the United States, all the guidelines on pain management emphasize that institutional approaches must be interdisciplinary to be most effective. Much of the emphasis on improving interdisciplinary approaches to pain management, therefore, has focused on promoting more effective teamwork between physicians and nurses. In this country, as in England and Canada, nurses have major responsibility for assessing and managing patients' pain, day to day, in most treatment settings. In other parts of the world, the role of nurses in pain assessment and management varies widely.[13]

> *In the United States, all the guidelines on pain management emphasize that institutional approaches must be interdisciplinary to be most effective. Much of the emphasis on improving interdisciplinary approaches to pain management, therefore, has focused on promoting more effective teamwork between physicians and nurses.*

Making pain the "fifth vital sign" on hospital charts on which temperature, pulse, respiration, and blood pressure are routinely recorded is now becoming more widespread in U.S. hospitals. The U.S. Veterans Administration health system recently adopted this as a systemwide policy.

In Europe, a similar campaign to improve pain management institution-wide, entitled *Vers un hôpital sans douleur,* is underway in several countries through the efforts of an international organization called *Association Internationale Ensemble Contre la Douleur*.[14] (See Appendix A: Targeted Resources and Tools, Part Three for the organization's website.) Many international pain and palliative care organizations have been working with the World Health Organization's Cancer Pain Relief Program to facilitate broad dissemination of its analgesic ladder and cancer pain guidelines.[15-17]

The practical aspects of implementing and measuring the effects of pain management guidelines on practice and on patient outcomes have not yet received much attention. In the interview that follows this editorial, Anna Du Pen, ARNP,

MN, and Stuart Du Pen, MD, provide insight into the effective use of an algorithm they developed that operationalizes the AHCPR guidelines on cancer pain management.[8] The algorithm, which is designed for use by physician–nurse teams, promotes better decision making about the treatment of pain at any stage in the cancer trajectory. The Du Pens discuss barriers to effective implementation of the algorithm and suggest ways to promote its use by both hospital-based oncology professionals and community-based providers.

In the International Perspectives section of this part, Michael Zenz, MD, an internationally recognized expert on pain management at BG University Clinic Bergmannsheil in Bochum, Germany, comments on the current state of pain management in his country. He advocates an interdisciplinary approach to pain assessment, diagnosis, and treatment from the first patient visit and a greater role for oncologists in the management of cancer pain.

ACKNOWLEDGMENT

I am grateful to my colleague Judith Spross, RN, PhD, director of the Mayday-PainLink initiative at the Education Development Center, Inc., for her substantive contributions to this editorial.

REFERENCES

1. Committee on Care at the End of Life, Institute of Medicine. *Approaching Death: Improving Care at the End of Life.* Washington, DC: National Academy Press, 1997, pp. 128-134.
2. Foley K. Pain assessment and cancer pain syndromes. In: Doyle D, Hanks GWC, MacDonald N, eds. *Oxford Textbook of Palliative Medicine,* 2nd ed. Oxford, United Kingdom: Oxford University Press, 1998, pp. 310-330.
3. Zenz M, Willweber-Strumpf A. Opiophobia and cancer pain in Europe. *Lancet* 1993;341:1075-1076.
4. Gordon DB. Critical pathways: A road to institutionalizing pain management. *J Pain Symptom Management.* 1996;11(4):252-259.
5. Spross J. "The Influence of Selected Societal, Institutional, and Individual Factors on Nurses' and Physicians' Pain Management Knowledge." [PhD dissertation, Boston College, 1999].
6. Max M. Improving outcomes of analgesic treatment: Is education enough? *Ann Int Med* 1990;113:885-889.
7. Bookbinder M, Coyle N, Kiss M, et al. Implementing national standards for cancer pain management: Program model and evaluation. *J Pain Symptom Management* 1996; 12(6):334-347.
8. Du Pen S, Du Pen AR, Polissar N, Hansberry J, Kraybill BM, Stillman M, Panke J, Everly R, Syrjala K. Implementing guidelines for cancer pain management: Results of a randomized controlled clinical trial. *J Clin Oncol* 1999;17(1):361-370.
9. American Pain Society. Quality improvement guidelines for the treatment of acute and cancer pain. *JAMA* 1995; 274(23):1874-1880.
10. Agency for Health Care Policy and Research. *Clinical Practice Guideline Number 9: Management of Cancer Pain* [AHCPR Publication No. 94-0592]. Rockville. MD: US

Department of Health and Human Services, Public Health Service, Agency for Health Care Policy and Research, 1994.

11. Oncology Nursing Society. Position statement: Cancer pain management. *Oncol Nurs Forum* 1998;25(5):817–818.

12. http://painconsult.com/MainPages/PatientLearning/NewsStand/Articles/JCAHO.html

13. *Cancer Pain Release* 1997;10(1):5–8.

14. Besner GF, Rapin, C-H. The hospital—creating a pain-free environment: A program to improve pain control in hospitalized patients. *J Palliative Care* 1993,9(1):51–52.

15. Foley KM. The World Health Organization Program in Cancer Pain Relief and Palliative Care. In: Gebhart, GI, Hammond DL, Jensen TS, eds. *Proceedings of the 7th World Congress on Pain: Progress in Pain Research and Management,* vol. 2. Seattle: IASP Press, 1994, pp. 59–74.

16. World Health Organization. *Cancer Pain Relief,* 2nd ed. Geneva: World Health Organization, 1996.

17. World Health Organization. *Cancer Pain Relief and Palliative Care.* Geneva: World Health Organization, 1990.

Designing and Implementing a Cancer Pain Algorithm

An Interview with ANNA DU PEN, ARNP, MN,
and STUART DU PEN, MD

*Swedish Medical Center
Seattle, Washington*

The Cancer Pain Algorithm is a step-by-step decision-tree model developed by Anna Du Pen, ARNP, MN, Stuart Du Pen, MD, and their colleagues at the Swedish Medical Center in Seattle, Washington, for use by physician–nurse oncology teams for treating patients suffering from cancer pain. This algorithm represents one attempt to operationalize the Clinical Practice Guideline Number 9: Management of Cancer Pain developed by the U.S. Agency for Health Care Policy and Research (AHCPR) [now called the Agency for Healthcare Research and Quality (AHRQ)]. This comprehensive pain-assessment and analgesic algorithm offers clinicians the opportunity to systematize their responses to patients suffering from cancer pain. The Du Pens and their colleagues have embarked on a series of educational interventions and research studies to implement and evaluate the efficacy of the ACHPR guidelines as they are activated through this algorithm. So far, these researchers have tested the algorithm in one randomized case-controlled study, which demonstrated that the algorithm does enhance patient pain outcomes.[2] Specifically, the researchers found that the oncology outpatients who were randomized to the treatment group did experience improved "usual" pain scores. In this phase 1 study, research teams of physicians and nurses implemented the algorithm for the treatment group of patients. In a second, as-yet-unpublished phase of this work, the researchers went on to train physician–nurse oncology teams to use the algorithm. In the following edited interview with Anna L. Romer, EdD, the Du Pens offer an overview of how the algorithm works and discuss what they have learned about the process of designing and implementing this pharmacologic decision-making process, including the challenges and barriers encountered in training others to implement it in outpatient oncology clinics.

PROBLEMS IN PRACTICE THAT LED TO DEVELOPMENT OF THE CANCER PAIN ALGORITHM

Stuart Du Pen: Why do we even have a protocol? Why did we set out to do this? It's not that nurses and physicians were doing a bad job *per se*. However, we made two important observations about practice and knowledge early on as we developed the algorithm: First, physicians would tend to simply grab the most recent drugs they had been using, and/or the ones they were most familiar with as their next choices to treat patients' pain. Clinicians—physicians and nurses—weren't tending to use the adjuvant drugs with their patients as extensively as the guidelines suggest is appropriate. Clinicians didn't really know when to use adjuvants, and, with opioids, when they should titrate the opioid up or move on to a different opioid, or which opioid would make a next-best choice.

There was no logical decision-making process that they could pull out and look at, and this is what led us to develop this decision-tree model. (See Figure 4.) We think that there should be a logical way that a clinician approaches a patient who has cancer-related pain and works through the system—an efficient method versus just "shooting in the dark." Treating pain gets confusing for clinicians, including oncologists. For example, when Mrs. Jones comes in with breast cancer and the tumor has spread to bone, and now we have movement-related pain, you think, "The pain's not controlled! Where do we go?"

The algorithm is a useful tool, even for clinicians like myself experienced in pain management. In my clinical practice, I may forget to apply certain segments and having a written algorithm I can look at quickly reminds me of my choices: "Oh, I didn't ask about the neuropathic part of it or the somatic part of it. I really should use a nonsteroidal anti-inflammatory; I haven't tried it." All of a sudden, the patient has dramatic pain relief because we've added these adjuvants. Now we don't have to fight through the high-dose narcotics as much and deal with narcotic barriers as much as we would had we just tried to cover [the pain] with a narcotic alone. So, having something to which you can refer back to remind you, the same way you do with antibiotics, is a real boon.

HOW THE ALGORITHM WORKS: KEY STEPS AND TOOLS

Anna L. Romer: *What triggers the algorithm and how does it work?*

Anna Du Pen: The nurses are trained that decision making flows from the asessment of the patient's pain. The day-to-day implementation of the algorithm is driven by a routine assessment of pain intensity and pain character. We have since added pain pattern, because there was such a divergence of effect between usual and worst pain in our first controlled study of the use of the algorithm. (Usual pain is "your pain level most of the time;" worst pain is "the worst your pain ever gets.") The practical implementation during the second study was that when the

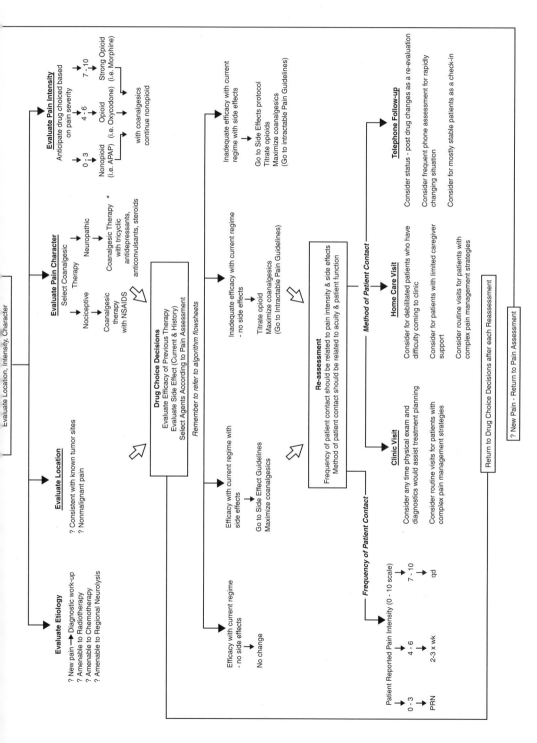

Figure 4. The Cancer Pain Algorithm

113

nurses had contact with the patients, whether it was a clinic visit, a phone triage, or a home-care visit, the first and most basic part of the interaction was to get a pain score on a scale of 0–10 as a measure of pain intensity. To measure pain character, we made a concise word list of nine words (burning, aching, stabbing, shooting, tender, dull, sharp, throbbing, and electric-like), just a bare-bones minimum number of words that patients could say, "Yes I have this one," or "It's shooting, and it's also aching." Our idea was that, although we have some extensive tools such as the Brief Pain Inventory (BPI) and the McGill-Melzack Scale, they're not feasible for practical, everyday use. So we really had to get it down to, "Is your pain controlled or not?" and "What kind of pain is it?" That answer leads us to the choice of coanalgesics. (See Figure 5. Pain-Assessment Routine) A step in this routine pain-assessment decision tree is to assess for the presence of side effects, such as constipation and oversedation. For each of the most common side effects, we've created a separate decision-tree tool.

Making the analgesic drug choices is a longitudinal process; there is no single intervention. We try out a particular medication, based on the algorithm, and then do a reassessment to check how it is working and cycle back through the process

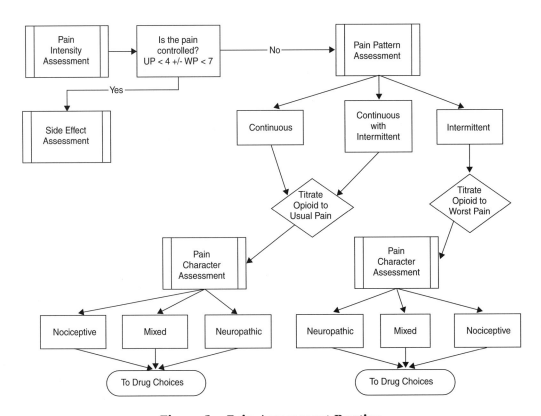

Figure 5. Pain Assessment Routine

This tool is part of the Cancer Pain Algorithm, Copyright ©1999 Du Pen, Inc. Reprinted here with permission from Anna and Stuart Du Pen.

of drug choice and side-effect evaluation after each reassessment, or revisit the basic pain assessment if new kinds of pain occur. (See Figure 6. Reassessment)

ALR: *Was this initial contact driven by the patient or by the study?*

ADP: In the phase 1 study, which was published in the *Journal of Clinical Oncology,*[2] the contact was driven by the study, because we were really trying to implement and validate the algorithm. And, as you know, when researcher physician–nurse teams implemented the algorithm, it did improve pain management for usual pain, as reported by patients. In the second phase, when we trained the providers, the doctors and nurses, then I think the algorithm was just driven by patient contact. This systematic pain assessment was generally not part of standard treatment.

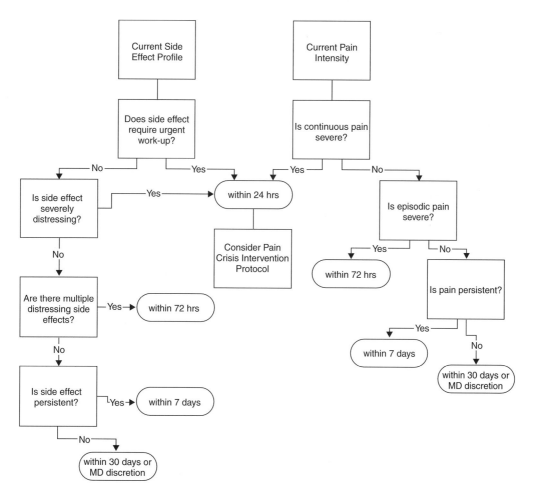

Figure 6.   Reassessment

This tool is part of the Cancer Pain Algorithm, Copyright ©1999 Du Pen, Inc. Reprinted here with permission from Anna and Stuart Du Penn.

MODELING THE INTERVENTION ON EXISTING PRACTICE PATTERNS

ADP: We were aware of several barriers that had to be overcome in order for the algorithm to be implemented efficiently into already-busy oncology outpatient clinics. We designed our training and tools to map onto existing systems so that clinicians, nurses, and physician teams, would recognize them as similar routines to what they already do but with a different content focus: pain. We used the analogy of chemotherapy treatment, because we felt that this would be comfortable for them.

We knew that for the implementation to work, nurses had to play a key role in operationalizing the algorithm. We are aware of process issues between nurses and doctors that can sometimes get in the way of best patient care, and we see these tools as a way to encourage teamwork for the benefit of the patient. These are not nurse documents or doctor documents; they are just short tools that could be used to tie together the work of the physicians and nurses.

During the one-day training in the phase 2 study, one of the ways the role-model consultants tried to bring that point home was by making an analogy to the chemotherapy protocol. In that protocol, the patients are seen in the laboratory for their blood work; they come to the nurse first, the evaluation of the laboratory work is done, and then the nurse goes to the doctor and says, "The white count is such and such. It looks like the protocol calls for a drop in the next dose of chemo." The doctor basically signs off on it. The nurse runs the medication order to the pharmacy, and the dose reduction is carried out, essentially all facilitated, in an operational sense, by the nurse. So, what the consultants tried to do in talking to the doctor-nurse teams was to say, "Look, this is just another component of care that is best optimized by having the nurse operationalize it, and here's the way it's done: The patient comes in, the patient gives a pain score that's very similar to a laboratory test, and the nurse comes to the doctor and says, 'Look, the patient's pain level is an 8, and the MSContin® is at 60, and the protocol calls for a 50 percent increase, which is the next dose that it would be, whatever that dose is. Is that all right with you? Can we go ahead and implement that?'" And the doctor signs off on it, because we still don't want to go so far in this automation of the process that the doctor is unable to use his or her judgment to make decisions based on the individual needs of the patient. But in a general sense, the care is optimized by having the protocol in the hands of the nurse.

> *We knew that for the implementation to work, nurses had to play a key role in operationalizing the algorithm. We are aware of process issues between nurses and doctors that can sometimes get in the way of best patient care, and we see these tools as a way to encourage teamwork for the benefit of the patient.*

ALR: *What other strategies did you use that were specifically geared to promoting the use of the algorithm and the cooperation of the physician–nurse team?*

ADP: We have a progress note and a flow chart. The flow chart was modeled after a chemotherapy flow chart. In other words, in most oncology clinics there's a flow chart that shows what chemotherapy drugs the patient is on, what the white count is, when the patient got the last dose. It's a regimented form that oncology clinicians are used to filling out. It's a kind of tracking form.

We tried to integrate a pain flow chart into that same form. In other words, we have a model flow chart, but we wanted to give each individual clinic the option of whether to use it as a separate form or to integrate it into their existing flow charts. Basically, what it showed was that, on the same date, right underneath the laboratory value, there's a pain score of 8, this is the medicine that the patient was on, this is the modification in medication that was made, and this is where we checked to see if there were any of the seven core side effects that we follow in the algorithm. So, we basically tried to integrate the use of the algorithm into the way the clinicians were already operating.

The progress note, which was designed as sort of a clinic checkoff, is a very concise one-page tool, and it says, "Is the pain controlled or not? Is the patient having side effects or not?"

That was done by the nurse, for the most part, because that's the assessment phase, where the two primary questions are: "Is the pain controlled or not?" and "Are they having side effects from their analgesics, yes/no?" At the bottom of that piece of the form, there is a treatment recommendation that has to be followed through by the doctor. Again, it's just a checkbox, "Optimize coanalgesics (check). Titrate opioids (check)." So, it's another communication device that ties the doctor and nurse together.

Some nurses told us they didn't feel comfortable going to the doctor and saying that we need to increase the MSContin® from 60 to 75 or from 60 to 90 or whatever the titration protocol suggested. They weren't comfortable in their own discipline recommending something to the doctor. So, we tried to take that into account by having the recommendation come from the document, the Cancer Pain Algorithm.

POTENTIAL BARRIERS TO CONSIDER WHEN TRAINING OTHERS TO IMPLEMENT THE ALGORITHM

Physician–Nurse Team Issues

ALR: *What makes physician–nurse teams work?*

SDP: Well, let me just say that the closest relationship between a physician and a nurse seems to be in oncology, much more so than in, say, urology or general surgery, where a nurse-practitioner or a nurse-partner is more in the office, dealing with new patients as they come in, are treated, and then leave; whereas, with oncology, the patient comes into the practice and is a long-term occupant of the practice. So, the physician and nurse play a much closer role, both with each other and with the patient and family. The oncology nurses follow individual patients within that physician–nurse practice and they know exactly where each patient is. The patient calls and talks to the nurse on a first-name basis, and they become very close. The nurses know who the relatives are; they become an integral part of that relationship. So, it's a much closer set of relationships among the physician, the nurse, the patient, and the patient's family than within the other types of practices, and it's very clearly related to the nature of the practice.

ADP: In my experience, that would be a really nice template if it were true for every oncology doctor and nurse but, unfortunately, I don't think it is. I think that the physician definitely drives the temperament of the interaction with the patient, and even if you have a wonderful nurse who is really into pain management, if the physician, for whatever reason, is one who believes that you can't treat the pain optimally because it will interfere with the antitumor treatment or diagnostic stuff, it doesn't happen.

During our one-day training in the phase 2 study, Michael Levy, Pam Kedziera, Vivian Scheidler, and Stuart Grossman—the consultants who served as role-model physician–nurse teams and trained the physician–nurse pairs—spent a lot of time trying to reinforce the idea that it was O.K. for the nurses to do some of the decision making. The algorithm is driven by assessment, even to the level of how much to titrate the opioid, and nurses are perfectly capable, and perhaps more in tune with the patients, to drive some of these protocols. So, I think there was some background in their minds, and probably also in my mind, that the physician has to be committed to the concepts of palliative medicine and has to be able to delegate some of the responsibility for moving the protocol along to the nurse.

In some cases it did work that way. In other cases, the nurses would say things like, "Well, he doesn't want me to make a recommendation . . . he wants to make all the decisions himself." Some nurses reported that physicians seemed to be intimidated when they used tools associated with the algorithm, such as equianalgesic charts to determine what the dose of the new drug should be. It seemed in those instances that control issues got in the way and that physicians who did not already have access to this knowledge found it intimidating in this form, that is, coming from the nurse. So, the response in those cases, as reported by nurses, was that the doctor wanted to have control of the dosage decision on his or her own—even though he or she didn't have this knowledge at his or her fingertips—without using the equianalgesic chart. That does happen, and I'm not sure what the best way to deal with that tension is.

Limitations of One-Day Training

SDP: We found that, when we trained clinicians to implement the algorithm, once we completed the teaching process, the patient outcomes only showed improved pain scores for the first four months after the training. Then the effects of the training seemed to wear off. The physician–nurse teams were back to doing the same things they were doing before the training.

We think this occurred because we taught them, but we didn't update the teaching. In phase 2, we wanted to determine what impact that one intensive day of teaching would have over time. So, purposefully, we gave tools to the participants, and we, as the researchers, remained available to them, but we didn't go back in and re-educate.

ADP: I think that we were hamstrung a bit by the clinical research format. But the benefits clearly are that the outcomes are improved when the process is implemented. The weaknesses are that unless you have a motivated learner, the one-shot teaching may not stick. We did notice the variability of interest and commitment among the clinicians we were training. One of the groups included a medical director of a hospice, who was obviously very interested in implementing this. Another group had some doctors that were totally uninterested in palliative care, yet, the nurses in the clinic were very interested and had the reference guide with them at their desks. Some of those things are nearly impossible to capture in terms of a research variable.

Organizational Barriers to Implementation

ADP: We noticed that implementation fell down in some individual clinics because of reorganization and systems issues. For example, in one clinic, we had a doctor–nurse team that was very strong. Both were very interested in palliative care to begin with and were clearly working hard to implement the algorithm. The way we knew that is because the progress notes were consistently done and were in the chart, which we knew because we were doing chart audits. Then the managed care organization where their clinic was located underwent major shifts in personnel and oversight. As a result, they lost one of the doctors out of the clinic and then the main nurse who was working with one of the doctors got ill and things just sort of fell apart there for several months, mainly because of lack of resources to follow through on the implementation.

"I Feel Like I'm Buried in Paperwork"

ADP: We surveyed the doctors and nurses at the end of participating in the study, and they gave us anecdotal feedback. One said, "You know, I just can't do the progress note, because I'm totally overwhelmed and at the end of the day, I literally feel like I'm buried in paperwork." So, the other issue here about why it may or may not work has to do with whether or not the resources are there to allow them to do such things as call back the patient and say, "Look, Mr. Jones, your pain was a 9 out of 10 two days ago or whatever and we made this change in your medicine . . . what's your pain score today?"

This brings us back to one of the key steps in the algorithm: the reassessment. The reassessment parameters say that if you have a patient with severe pain, that patient needs to have some sort of checkback in 24 hours. So, if a patient comes in with a 9 out of 10 pain score, you implement some sort of recommendation from the algorithm, and you have a checkback the next day. We tried to encourage the nurses either to ask the patients to call them or to call the patients themselves, depending on how the system was best going to work for that practice.

But we found that although the checkback would happen, it would not happen for a week. Actually, we were gratified that it happened in a week, because we were fearful that, had it not been for the algorithm, that contact probably would not have been made at all because there was an overwhelming sense among the nurses of just needing to get through their days, to give the anti-tumor therapy, which was the first priority.

WAYS TO ADDRESS THESE BARRIERS

ADP: Two things are going to help with implementing a system or a process in an institution where people lack motivation in the area or feel they don't have time to do the paperwork and follow through. First, as you are probably well aware, the Joint Commission on Accreditation of Healthcare Organizations has been moving toward including pain assessment and management standards for accreditation. That will be the big hammer—to mandate that processes like this be instituted.

Second, we're trying to move more toward an automated system, which can be easily updated. We have another grant from the National Cancer Institute to transfer the knowledge into a computerized decision-support system that will take pain-assessment data and generate treatment recommendations. We're hoping that this electronic tool will reinforce implementation of the algorithm, because if the algorithm is not used, then it obviously doesn't work!

PATIENT "NONADHERENCE" IN THE FACE OF PAIN AND NO MEDICATION SIDE EFFECTS

ALR: *In your first paper, you observed that some patients refused to take prescribed treatments even when pain was not well controlled and there were no side effects. What did the researcher physicians and nurses do in those cases?*

ADP: We were actually surprised that it was such a problem. About one out of three patients refused to take the prescribed medications. We went into this with the idea that, if we had the ability to educate patients and make sure they understood the medicines they were taking, made sure they understood things like fear of addiction, and made sure side effects were tracked and treated aggressively because we knew side effects were a major barrier, then we would be able to see much less nonadherence in the group treated using the algorithm versus those patients receiving standard treatment.

What we found is that there were some pretty major barriers to patient adherence that we didn't have a good grip on before we went into this. One of them definitely was the cost of the medication. Patients reported to us that they were actually rationing their pills because of the cost of the pills. We were saying to patients, "Make sure that, if you feel the pain coming on, you take the medicine before the pain gets too bad, because it's easier to treat the pain beforehand than to treat it after it's out of control." That's one of our standard patient teaching messages. What we discovered, however, in talking to some of these people was that their decision making about when to take their pills had less to do with our instructions—even when they understood our instruction to take their medicine preemptively—than with how much money they had to spend on their pills versus groceries or rent.

Patients Who Say, "I Don't Want To"

A second barrier to following the algorithm was a particular stance some patients took toward taking the recommended medicines, what we began to call the "I-don't-want-to" group. This was a substantial group of patients. What we found is that people in this group are just anti-pill. When you talk to these people, you can explain the situation about the narcotic medicines not being dangerous or addictive and you can explain about the implications of unrelieved pain, which are pretty drastic. For example, we know a lot now about the fact that unrelieved pain compromises the immune system. So, we have a lot of powerful teaching tools, yet the patients would tell us things like, "Ever since I was a young kid, I've tried to stay away from pills. I just don't like pills. I don't want to take pills. It's O.K., I'll just have some pain; I'd rather have the pain than take the pills."

Other clinicians and researchers would tell us, "Well, that's just an educational problem." But you know, in phase 1, we had three full-time nurses who did nothing but interact with these patients and educate them, to an extent that would not be feasible in terms of what can normally occur in a clinic. I mean, it's just not feasible for three nurses to be working on nothing but pain management. So, we're pretty confident that we covered the education piece pretty solidly. Even so, some patients, although fully informed about the medication, still said, "I don't want to."

> *A second barrier to following the algorithm was a particular stance some patients took toward taking the recommended medicines, what we began to call the "I-don't-want-to" group. This was a substantial group of patients. What we found is that people in this group are just anti-pill. When you talk to these people, you can explain the situation about the narcotic medicines not being dangerous or addictive and you can explain about the implications of unrelieved pain, which are pretty drastic, yet the patients would tell us things like, "Ever since I was a young kid, I've tried to stay away from pills. I just don't like pills. I don't want to take pills. It's O.K., I'll just have some pain; I'd rather have the pain than take the pills."*

The reality is that we need to address these issues in a very patient-centric way. You do that by asking patients what they do use for their pain or what else they would like to pursue in pain management if they're anti-pill.

Integrating Nonpharmacological Types of Pain Management

ADP: There is room for the nonpharmacological types of pain management, there is room for more complementary care, herbal remedies, and so on. Some patients are going to alternative care providers to get herbal remedies or something that is more "natural." Many, many times, patients would say to us, "We want something that's more natural." And some patients wanted to try other strategies, such as stress management, relaxation and imagery, physiotherapy, or heating pads. Some patients said, "If I have a choice of taking a pill or running to the store to buy a heating pad, I'm going to try the heating pad first."

Many times, it wasn't necessarily that they were anti-pill to the point where they weren't going to take any pills; it's just that they would prefer to do other things prior to doing that. And when we went to measure patient adherence, of course, we were measuring it against the algorithm, which said things like, "If you're beginning to feel an escalation of pain, take the pill early." This recommendation is supported by the evidence-based literature, which suggests that it may take more pain medicine to reduce the pain if one waits to take the pill. But, for the patient, the choice did not follow that line of reasoning. Such a patient would be labeled as less adherent according to this algorithm, even if in fact that patient did eventually take the pill after trying the heating pad.

This observation contributes to our constant revision of how we're measuring things. With respect to the algorithm—which, of course, is a pharmacological tool—we can only comment on patients' adherence to the drug therapy. In fact, we've looked at, and are still looking at, complementary techniques and non-pharmacological techniques and how they fit in. We did ask patients about this, and we have lots of data on whether or not they were using alternative or complementary techniques but, from a research perspective, it's not possible to factor those things in and still call patients "drug-adherent." So, we gathered more data as a means of explaining the factors that patients use to determine whether or not they will take their medicines. That will be the subject of another paper we plan to write on patient adherence, in which we will look at factors used by patients to determine whether or not they want to take their medicines.

For purposes of implementing the algorithm, I think this means that not only do we have to deal with institutional issues that create roadblocks to implementing the process, not only do we have to figure out a way to really help clinicians retain and continue to use the process, but we also have to recognize that the algorithm is just a tool to help bolster the patient–provider interface. We still have to come back and say, "We're in the business of patient-centric care." We recognize that patients will make decisions, and we absolutely want to make sure that they're educated about their medications, about pain and the implications of unrelieved pain; but ultimately (and I'm speaking for both of us, I think), we are in favor of patient-centric pain management.

Ongoing Negotiation Between Patient and Clinician Understandings

SDP: It truly becomes a negotiation. I find certain patients will accept, for example, Kadian, which is a long-acting, 24-hour morphine, when they don't want to take as many pills. Or they'll take a Duragesic® patch, because it isn't a pill and it's a different way of getting medication.

Moreover, the patient has a personal algorithm that may be different from the one we are using. We often try to get the patient to fit into our understanding of the process of prostate cancer, for example—what's going to happen to that patient in the long term, it's widely metastatic, that patient is going to die—but let's try to make him or her as comfortable as possible. Well, a patient's algorithm is: "I'm not going to die. This next chemotherapy is going to cure the problem. I'm going to be out skydiving like I've done before, or rock climbing, and this is where I'm going. I'm not going along your pattern that you're planning for me." So, it does become a real negotiation with the patient as to what medications the patient is willing to accept, because that patient's plan for the future is totally different from ours.

REASSESSMENT OF PAIN AS A MEANS TO RENEGOTIATE MEDICATION OPTIONS

ADP: The idea of an algorithm is not that 100 percent of the time, if you follow this box by an arrow to another box, then you will have the golden answer to the problem. From the perspective of the algorithm, the reassessment component probably speaks most to the idea of continuing to keep the patient in the loop. That is, you assess the patient, you elect a logical choice of pain medicine therapy, and then you always go back to the patient and ask, "Is the pain controlled? Are you having side effects?" And, generally speaking, the answer to one of those two questions will lead you into some renegotiation with the patient.

It's very flexible. You say to the patient, "I hear you're still having pain, but you're not having side effects and you've been taking your medicine only 30 percent of the time. My next step, according to the algorithm, would be to increase the medicine or change to a different medicine or add an adjuvant, but I need to know why you're not taking your pills so, together, we can take the next step in the algorithm and decide about either changing the drug or adding a second drug so that you don't need as much of the first drug."

The patient may say, "I'm only taking 30 percent of my medication because I want to use the heating pad and drink my chamomile tea, because I think that they're better for me." So, at some point, you try to say, "Well, let's explore why you think that. Is it because you're afraid of becoming addicted?" If so, you try to deal with it.

Or that patient may say, "No, I don't have any trouble taking the pill. I understand that it's O.K. to take the pill. I just prefer to do these other things." That response isn't necessarily anathema to the algorithm, because you're still doing the reassessment component, you're still monitoring the patient's pain level, you're still continuing to offer options to the patient; but at some point you listen to the patient and say, "O.K. You're going to do your heating pad, you're going to do your chamomile tea. On the occasions that you do choose to take the medication, let's see if there isn't a better way that you can gain more efficacy from the medicine during that 30 percent of the time that you're taking it." So, you try to utilize the logic and knowledge of the algorithm in the space where the patient is ready for you to do that.

CULTURAL DIVERSITY AND THE APPLICABILITY OF THE ALGORITHM

ALR: *Were there any issues connected to cultural diversity related to patient adherence to pain medication?*

SDP: The big key is the assessment and reassessment process, which I think would work fine in any ethnic environment.

ADP: We do not have large minority populations in the Seattle area, so we did not have enough patients from culturally diverse backgrounds to explore issues related to ethnicity. However, we do have a fair number of Pacific Islanders and a large population of Scandinavians, Norwegians and Swedes, in a subgroup in Seattle. At the risk of stereotyping, I would say that the Scandinavians can be incredibly stubborn and stoic and comprise a big part of the "I-don't-want-to" group of our patients. Among the Scandinavians is an attitude that pain is an obligatory part of the experience: "I can tough it out; I can get through this and it's a part of what I have to go through."

After the first part of the study, we did begin to ask patients what an acceptable level of pain was, because we heard so many patients saying, "No, I don't take the pain medicine until the pain gets to a certain level." We were surprised by how high the pain had to get before some patients would consider medication. I'd have to go back and look specifically at this, but some of these patients would say, "I don't take a pill until it gets to 7 out of 10 because I'm just determined to win over this pain." Or, "I am tough enough to put up with it." In my opinion, that definitely is a cultural kind of decision-making process.

DEVELOPING NEW TOOLS FOR PATIENT EDUCATION

ADP: Some of the other things we're currently doing with the algorithm include trying to develop good handouts for patient education and support so that in the event—as is the case many times—that the doctors or even the nurses are not skilled at being able to work through differences with their patients about pain medication, they will have some tools to use. I'm thinking specifically of information that's been coming out about unrelieved pain and the immune system, because it speaks directly to that "I'm-going-to-be-tough, I'm-going-to-fight-this-cancer" attitude. As a matter of fact, unless your pain is relieved, your body is not able to do its best work at fighting the cancer.

ALR: *Did you find that when a nurse actually explained this to patients that it affected their adherence to the treatment recommendations of the algorithm?*

ADP: In this study, we weren't measuring the patient-level outcomes of the educational intervention component. Basically, our feeling is that patient education is a component of what the nurse does as a part of the process of implementing the algorithm. But, just anecdotally, I can tell you that many times it does work. For example, in the general category of fear of addiction, people are misinformed, sometimes by their own doctors, which is kind of alarming. But the fear of addiction can and often is worked through fairly quickly; it doesn't have to be a 45-minute discussion.

INTERNATIONAL APPLICABILITY OF THE CANCER PAIN ALGORITHM

ALR: *Is your algorithm capable of adoption in countries where different drugs are used or available or where morphine is difficult to obtain?*

SDP: Yes, because we give options. We've got to give options to the doctor-nurse teams because they have different drugs and they tend to use different drugs. In Australia, we found, there is no Dilaudid® or hydromorphone available, and they were just getting the Duragesic® patch, the fentanyl patch. So, yes, there are differences, yet you can still use the algorithm. At the reassessment step, in which you are talking about titration of the opioid, clinicians can use whatever sort of opioid they have available.

When we were lecturing in Australia, we found that we had very little problem because alternative drugs are available. In China, on the other hand, where morphine is very restricted, that would pose a major problem for implementing the algorithm there.

ADP: Sometimes clinicians in other countries have more and sometimes they have fewer options than we have. In Australia, for example, they have nasal fentanyl, which we don't have. So, in some cases, they may have drugs that are better than the drugs we have, or they may add to the list of the ones we have. In some cases, the list of available agents will change. I think what we're emphasizing here is that it is not necessarily the availability of one or more of the drugs by themselves. It's really the process that's important. In a country where they don't have access to opioids at all, I think it would be much more difficult to implement the algorithm, but as long as there is some access to drugs in these categories, they can be used and combined in the process.

REFERENCES

1. Agency for Health Care Policy and Research. *Clinical Practice Guideline Number 9: Management of Cancer Pain* (AHCPR Publication No. 94-0592). Rockville, MD: U.S. Department of Health and Human Services, Public Health Services, Agency for Health Care Policy and Research, 1994.
2. Du Pen S, Du Pen AR, Polissar N, Hansberry J, Kraybill BM, Stillman M, Panke J, Everly R, Syrjala K. Implementing guidelines for cancer pain management: Results of a randomized controlled clinical trial. *J Clin Oncol* 1999;17(1):361–370.

Some Thoughts on Pain Management in Germany

An Interview with MICHAEL ZENZ, MD

BG University Clinic, Bergmannsheil
Bochum, Germany

During an interview with Anna L. Romer, EdD, Michael Zenz, MD, director of Anaesthesiology, Intensive Care and Pain Therapy at BG University Clinic, Bergmannsheil, in Bochum, Germany comments on the current state of pain management in his country.

Anna L. Romer: *What is most needed in Germany now to provide good pain management for patients near the end of life?*

Michael Zenz: In Germany, the greatest need is simply symptom control. We are highly deficient in just doing good pain control for those patients. Also, we actually have no place for patients whose cure-oriented treatment fails. We are not allowed to keep these patients in our hospitals. So, if surgery fails, or if pills and chemotherapy fail, we are not allowed to hold the patients longer in the hospital, and yet we do not have enough palliative care places, nor enough institutions that provide home care, and we simply have no idea what to do with these patients. We have hospices, but not at all enough. For example, in my town of Bochum, which has a population of 500,000, we have a hospice with only eight beds. I have a huge outpatient pain clinic, but I have only six inpatient beds, certainly not enough to serve those people who need round-the-clock care in a town the size of Bochum. It's impossible.

ALR: *So what happens to people who are dying in pain?*

MZ: They are left to the random opportunities afforded by their environments. It just depends on the family, on whether there is a pain clinician in the neighborhood, or an exceptional oncologist, who knows how to provide modern pain therapy. The problem is how to control pain at the moment, because more than 50 percent of patients in the different towns in Germany are not aware of any pain clinics. They are not referred to clinics. They are not contacted by a pain specialist. The home physicians have great difficulty in referring patients to pain a specialists because they are upset about losing their patients, and so forth.

ALR: *How many pain clinics exist in Germany?*

MZ: About 50, and there are about 250 pain specialists.

ALR: *What, in your view, are the main issues or problems with pain and symptom management in Germany?*

MZ: I think, in my context, as in most others, the main problem is the lack of an interdisciplinary approach to pain therapy. By interdisciplinary, I mean that, from the point of first contact with the patient through the last period of treatment, several disciplines are involved concomitantly in diagnosing and treating the patient's pain. Pain is not simply a biological problem, but also a biosocial/psychological problem, so the diagnosis and treatment of pain should include all those dimensions, both for cancer and noncancer pain. For example, at the first meeting with a patient in our clinic, I see the patient together with a psychologist, a neurologist, and a physiotherapist, and together we come to a conclusion about the diagnosis and course of treatment. This interdisciplinary approach to the treatment of pain is already accepted here for patients who are receiving palliative care, insofar as palliative medicine includes not only pain therapy, but also social, spiritual, and psychological support of the patient and family. It includes within its scope contact with the family, attention to the patient's environment, and so forth. The same should be true for every patient with chronic pain, for whom the influences from outside are certainly important to consider in making a diagnosis and planning therapy.

ALR: *Is your interdisciplinary approach to pain management typical in Germany?*

MZ: No, it is not typical. But it should be, worldwide.

ALR: *How have you been able to create this innovative type of practice in your setting?*

MZ: It has happened over time. I started as a single anesthetist doing pain therapy, and over time it became more and more obvious that whoever is performing pain therapy, whether anesthetists or interns or neurologists or whatever, they are limited in what they can do by their particular disciplinary focus on the one side, and by the complex needs of the patient, who has more than just the wish for injections or some painkillers, on the other side. It soon became obvious that pain therapy should involve more than one discipline. So to start with we employed psychologists, and then, as a second step, physiologists and physiotherapists, and as a third step, neurologists as regular and always-present members of our pain clinic staff.

ALR: *What role do nurses play on the pain management team?*

MZ: There are relatively few university-trained nurses in this country, and their role in pain management teams is very limited. Although the role of nurses is certainly accepted in Germany, in general, pain therapy in this country traditionally has been very far removed from nurses. That is an effect of financial pressures, legal constraints, and educational barriers. We do not pay physicians, nurses, or psychologists separately. We are paid per consultation or per injection. We receive a certain amount of money per visit, no matter how many clinicians are involved. This system of payment leads to different decisions about whom to engage in the care of the patient. Most colleagues do not include nurses in the outpatient treatment setting, but take on the nursing role themselves. Naturally, nurses do play a role in patient care at inpatient clinics, but we do not have specially trained nurses. The nurses who work in the inpatient pain clinic are nurses from the surgical or internal medicine ward working together with us, the pain specialists.

ALR: *In your setting, who does that initial assessment of pain? What sets in motion your first meeting with a patient?*

MZ: It is always a physician, in our clinic or outside our clinic. By law, treatment for pain can only be initiated by a physician's order. I am only allowed to treat when another physician refers a patient to me. We have no allowance to treat when a nurse thinks interdisciplinary pain therapy would be beneficial for the patient.

This system works well, because our traditions are different from the American traditions. The position of nurses is completely different in Germany than in the United States. For example, we don't have registered nurses. But this is changing in your direction. We are just beginning to establish university training for nurses. The first nursing professors were instituted in Germany only one or two years ago.*

ALR: *Are algorithms, or step-by-step decision-making tools like the decision tree that the Du Pens describe in* Innovations *commonly used for pain and symptom assessment and management in Germany?*

MZ: Yes, certainly, but more in areas outside the cancer pain arena, such as back pain, headache, or reflex sympathetic dystrophy. For cancer pain, the WHO [World Health Organization] Analgesic Ladder is more or less accepted in Germany, with some institutions discussing the implementation of steps before and after that ladder, but there are no algorithms like the Du Pens' algorithm for cancer pain in Germany.

ALR: *Would it be helpful to use such an algorithm, do you think, in your country?*

MZ: I think it would be helpful, but again, the situation is different from that in

---

*For an overview of the efforts to improve cancer pain management and palliative care among nurses internationally, see the entire issue of *Cancer Pain Release* 1997;10(1). In particular, see selected abstracts from different national perspectives in Research in Cancer Pain and Palliative Care: Part 1: Assessing Needs in Pain and Palliative Nursing Education (pp. 5–6) and Part 2: Interventions to Improve Pain and Palliative Nursing Education (pp. 7–8).

the United States because in Germany, the different disciplines involved in the treatment of cancer patients are still fighting a little bit about who cancer pain treatment should "belong" to. The major camps in this debate are the pain therapists and the oncologists. Oncology in Germany is more or less chemotherapy and not pain therapy. So, as an example, we do not have a single university department of oncology to which a palliative medicine ward is connected. We have palliative medicine in Germany but in no case is it connected to a university department of oncology. Oncologists here just focus on treating the patient in a curative sense, but not in a palliative sense.

In England, for example, the tradition is completely different. As you know, the English have several chairs of palliative medicine, whereas we in Germany have none. Certainly, there is much progress needed in this area in my country. To divide oncology from palliative medicine, in my opinion, misunderstands the actual situation of people with cancer. I think oncology and palliative medicine belong to each other and should never be divided in two different parts. Oncologists should be specialists in pain therapy as well as in cancer treatment, but at the moment they are not.

ALR: *How is pain managed near the end of life for patients with diseases other than cancer, for example, for patients with HIV or for very elderly people?*

MZ: In Germany, the public discussion of appropriate care near the end of life is still a little bit limited just to cancer patients. Certainly, the HIV and geriatric populations present situations similar to cancer patients. With respect to HIV, that's an area where, worldwide, there are deficits in treating those patients sufficiently when they develop pain, in part due to prejudices and myths still present in the public and among the health care professionals.

ALR: *What are the main barriers to good pain control in your context?*

MZ: That is a very, very difficult point because it is certainly hard to understand for people who don't know the social situation in Germany. I think there are many barriers. One is that pain therapy, if performed scientifically and correctly, makes no money in Germany at the moment. To give you an example, I make my living from being an anesthesiologist, not from managing pain in our clinic, which runs up a fortune in deficits each year. That is due to the fact that the services of three, four, or five colleagues, all working at the same time with the same patient are reimbursed at a rate of only $10 an hour, or something like that.

Interdisciplinary pain management is not reimbursed. What is reimbursed, and what you can live off very nicely, is making injections. But in my opinion, just to say, "Where does it hurt?" and then point to where it hurts and give an injection is not pain therapy.

Another barrier is that we have no systematic education about pain management taught at the medical universities; pain therapy is not part of our curriculum. We have ten questions about pain therapy on the exam, but no course on pain therapy as a required part of the education of our medical students. We also have no education on pain for specialists in other disciplines—oncologists, for example. So, in Germany, pain management is something for enthusiasts and not for people who have been educated properly.

In addition, legal and regulatory concerns are a very severe obstruction to providing good pain management because the prescription forms for opioids are very, very tough in Germany. The officials are very tough, physicians are penalized when we make mistakes on the prescriptions, and so forth.

ALR: *Does that make physicians afraid of prescribing opioids?*

MZ: Certainly. That's a big barrier. For example, we did an investigation of how pain was managed in more than 300 practices of internal and general practitioners in Germany for the years 1990–1993. Out of the more than 16,000 patients with a histologic diagnosis of cancer treated in those practices, only 327 received a prescription of morphine in a period of 3 years. Ninety-eight percent of the patients never received any morphine over that period!

After that investigation, the German government made an inquiry to general practitioners and practitioners of internal medicine, which had some very interesting results. For example, 97 percent of the doctors said, "Yes, the WHO Analgesic Ladder is a valuable ladder, and we do need step number three [morphine] of that ladder." Some pages later on in the questionnaire, there was the question, "Do you need morphine for your treatment?" The same 97 percent said, "No! I never need morphine!" They first say, "Yes, I do accept the WHO Analgesic Ladder, including morphine," and some questions later they say, "No, I never need morphine." That is the situation in Germany among general practitioners and home physicians.

ALR: *It sounds as though there's an enormous gap in practice among the pain specialists, anesthesiologists, and the general practitioners understanding of how to treat cancer pain in Germany.*

MZ: They are centuries apart.

ALR: *Is the use of morphine much more common among anesthesiologists and pain specialists?*

MZ: It is much more accepted, certainly. However, we learned from an inquiry we made among doctors who specialize in pain therapy that 50 percent of them don't have the prescription forms to prescribe morphine—fifty percent of the specialists!

ALR: *To what do you attribute this?*

MZ: They fear the legal restrictions and possible punishment for prescribing it; it is something special, and they just don't do it.

ALR: *Given those circumstances, how do you explain your own quite distinct practice? What allows you to be different?*

MZ: Just experience. My belief in morphine is based on many years of good experiences. Morphine is the safest drug of the WHO essential drug list. This is my belief. There is not a single drug in the world that is safer than morphine when it's given according to scientific knowledge . . . by the clock, by mouth, by the ladder.

> *It would be innovative just to treat morphine as any other drug and say that everybody can prescribe it on the regular prescription form for any antibiotic or aspirin or whatever. Progress would be to accept that pain is an illness and not a symptom. Progress would be to include pain within the scope of the various disciplines, so cancer pain would be part of the focus of oncology.*

ALR: *What would be innovative in pain and symptom management in Germany right now?*

MZ: There are many points for innovation. It would be innovative just to treat morphine as any other drug and say that everybody can prescribe it on the regular prescription form for any antibiotic or aspirin or whatever. Progress would be to accept that pain is an illness and not a symptom. Progress would be to include pain within the scope of the various disciplines, so cancer pain would be part of the focus of oncology. Back pain should be seen as an illness and not a symptom and be the subject for neurosurgery or orthopedics, and so forth. Progress would be to generally and regularly educate students about pain, to regularly educate specialists about pain. One of the most important points for me is to establish chairs of pain, to establish chairs of palliative medicine in medical universities. For example, I hold a chair of anesthesiology, intensive care, and pain therapy. That was the first chair where pain therapy was included in Germany.

ALR: *How was that instituted?*

MZ: I was elected as an anesthesiologist to the University of Bochum. When I was deciding whether to come to Bochum, I said I would accept the position only if the University would change the chair of anesthesiology to be anesthesiology and pain. So the University did. It depends very much on the single person and the single initiative.

I think a few institutions in Germany have a little more experience in the development of an interdisciplinary approach to pain, as I said in the beginning. That is not generally true for Germany but for some institutions it is true. I think that is a point where perhaps others could learn from our experience. It costs a great deal of money, time, and effort to treat pain in an interdisciplinary way, but without that, I think it's worse for the patient, for the society, for everybody. It makes more sense to treat a patient collaboratively with other specialists from the very beginning rather than consecutively.

ALR: *In those places in Germany where the interdisciplinary approach to pain has been established, what has accounted for it? Is it the strength of personality of the people involved? Or, is it different compensation methods in those places?*

MZ: I think it is a combination of factors. Of course, it depends on the persons doing it, but I think more important is the clinical experience of those providers, of being involved in pain therapy over many years—and seeing not just cancer patients, because in cancer patients, the problems of providing interdisciplinary care are not as big as for many other patients. For example, in patients with low-back pain, you learn with experience that a somatic approach alone is almost never successful and, if you can, from the very beginning, start with what I think is the correct interdisciplinary treatment, you will be more effective and save time and effort.

ALR: *So, working across the spectrum of pain presentations, not just with patients near the end of life, allows you to see an approach that works better for all?*

MZ: Yes. It would certainly be true for those patients who need spiritual support, social support, and psychological support—all things that are self-evident in palliative medicine. There is no really good palliative care institution without a priest, a psychologist, a social worker, and so forth. So, that is certainly true for dying patients. But the problems are more evident for the patients with back pain and with headache and with reflex sympathetic dystrophy, because the interdisciplinary approach is largely absent in the treatment of noncancer, nonterminal pain.

ALR: *Do you see any changes taking place?*

MZ: I was a solo fighter some 15–20 years ago, and the topic keeps me fighting still. I think we will overcome the problem over the years. We've made great progress, although for you, as an American, the figures may sound very strange. But we have made huge progress. When I started as a pain clinician, I was only allowed to prescribe morphine for one single day—so the patient had to come to my clinic every day for a single-day prescription. Now we have prescription forms for 30 days. So, it's increased from 1 day, to 7 days, to 14 days, to, now, 30 days, and now, in special cases, we can prescribe for even longer periods than 30 days.

I see other dramatic changes. For example, we are one of the first countries in the world with an official specialization in pain therapy. That is new and is certainly a step in the right direction, but at the moment we are disputing with the officials about where to train these specialists, in which units, and which units are certified to train them.

ALR: *Would these pain specialists be affiliated with a pain clinic or with palliative care?*

MZ: More likely a pain clinic. In Germany, there is a division between palliative care and pain therapy; they do not automatically belong to each other. We have specialists who exclusively do palliative care and do not treat people who are not terminally ill, but who suffer from backache or headache. And we have pain therapists who treat backache or headache but do absolutely no palliative care.

I think it would be ideal if a specialist would have knowledge in both areas, but I accept that we need to institute pain clinics without palliative care for the vast majority of chronic pain patients, those with nonterminal and noncancer pain.

ALR: *One of the things that the Du Pens and others have observed in working with patients suffering from pain, especially near the end of life, is how important the side effects of medication can be in affecting people's adherence to pain treatment regimens. Can you comment on this issue from your experience?*

MZ: In our setting, we meet regularly with patients, every day, every second day or every week, until they are free of side effects and until the therapy can be followed up by the general physician at home. So, when we institute a certain therapy, which has side effects, we don't discharge the patient from the care of providers in our outpatient ambulatory clinic before the side effects are under control. We manage the pain level, the side effects, and the patient's vigilance in taking the medication as prescribed, and when everything is O.K., we can leave the patient to the care of the general physician.

ALR: *Do you have patients that resist taking opioids because they are afraid of becoming addicted?*

MZ: Yes, certainly we have. We have made an investigation into what happened at home when we prescribed opioids to patients. The results of that study prompted our decision to only discharge a patient to the care of the general practitioner when we know everything is O.K. What happened is, the patient went home and, at the first step, family members said, "Don't take morphine. That is dangerous." When this was overcome, the pharmacists said, "Oh! You shouldn't take morphine. Don't do that. I'll give you some aspirin. That is better." And so forth. So, we have prejudices everywhere, with the family, the pharmacist, the patient, and the whole environment, and we have to overcome these prejudices.

ALR: *How do you get the patient to believe you rather than these other people?*

MZ: There is no certain procedure. It is just talking to the patient. I tell patients to just try it, and if what I'm telling them is not true we can meet again next week or in two weeks, and they can tell me I was not right. So, I don't think it's a problem between the patient and me; it is a problem between the patient and his or her social environment.

ALR: *How do you overcome that?*

MZ: By regularly meeting with those patients on an outpatient basis until we know the treatment plan is running well, and that the pharmacist, the family, and the general practitioner, are accepting of the treatment plan as well. We speak to the family, we call the general practitioner, and we call the pharmacist. We speak with the patient about his or her fears and prejudices. Then we explain the side effects of medications and how we plan to treat them. We explain, for example, that nausea becomes less and less severe after two or three weeks of treatment. In this way, we try to enlist the patient's confidence in the treatment and how it will affect the patient's quality of life. We do not have any algorithms on this topic in Germany. We are not in the same place as you are in the United States, when it comes to cancer pain relief, but I think we are moving in the right direction. My colleagues and I wrote a piece a few years ago that still provides an accurate picture of the situation in Germany.[1]

REFERENCE

1. Zenz M, Zenz T, Tryba M, Strumpf M. Severe undertreatment of cancer pain: A 3-year survey of the German situation. *J Pain Symptom Management* 1995;10(3):187–191.

Selected Bibliography

Part Four

Selected articles by contributors to this part:

Du Pen S, Du Pen AR, Polissar N, Hansberry J, Kraybill BM, Stillman M, Panke J, Everly R, Syrjala K. Implementing guidelines for cancer pain management: Results of a randomized controlled clinical trial. *J Clin Oncol* 1999;17(1):361–370.

Du Pen SL, Williams AR. The dilemma of conversion from systemic to epidural morphine: A proposed conversion tool for treatment of cancer pain. *Pain* 1994;56(1):113–118.

Du Pen SL, Williams AR, Feldman RK. Epidurograms in the management of patients with long-term epidural catheters. *Regional Anesthesia* 1996;21(1):61–67.

Strumpf M, Zenz M, Donner B. Germany: Status of cancer pain and palliative care. *J Pain Symptom Management* 1996;12(2):109–111.

Zenz M. Pain therapy only for specialists or general responsibility [German] *Z Arztl Fortbild Qualitatissich* 1998;92(1):3

Zenz M, Willweber-Strumpf A. Opiophobia and cancer pain in Europe. *Lancet* 1993;341:1075–1076.

Zenz M, Zenz T, Tryba M, Strumpf M. Severe undertreatment of cancer pain: A 3-year survey of the German situation. *J Pain Symptom Management* 1995;10(3):187–191.

Other selected literature:

Agency for Health Care Policy and Research. *Clinical Practice Guideline: Management of Cancer Pain* [AHCPR Publication No. 94-0592]. Rockville, MD: U.S. Department of Health and Human Services, Public Health Services, Agency for Health Care Policy and Research, 1994.
(For print copies, contact AHCPR Publications Clearinghouse, P.O. Box 8547, Silver Spring, MD 20907; or call (800) 358-9295. A hypermedia presentation of the guideline is available online at: *www.talaria.org*)

American Pain Society. *Principles of Analgesic Use in the Treatment of Acute Pain and Cancer Pain,* 4th ed. Glenview, IL: American Pain Society, 1999.

Carr DB, Addison RG. *Pain in HIV/AIDS.* Washington, DC: France-USA Pain Association. 1994.

Colleau SM, Joranson DE. Fear of addiction: Confronting a barrier to cancer pain relief. *Cancer Pain Release* 1998;11(3):1–4,8.

Farber S, Anderson W, Bramden C, Isenhower P, Lanier K, O'Reilly L. Improving cancer pain management through a system wide commitment. *J Palliative Med* 1998;1(4):377–385.

Ferrell BR, Dean GE, Grant M, Coluzzi P. An institutional commitment to pain management. *J Clin Oncol* 1995;13(9):2158–2165.

Fins JJ. Acts of omission and commission in pain management: The ethics of naloxone use. *J Pain Symptom Management* 1999;17(2):120-124.

Foley K. A 44-year-old woman with severe pain at the end of life. *JAMA* 1999;81(20):1937-1945.

Foley KM. The World Health Organization Program in Cancer Pain Relief and Palliative Care. In: Gebhart GI, Hammond DL, Jensen TS, eds. *Proceedings of the 7th World Congress on Pain: Progress in Pain Research and Management,* vol. 2, Seattle, WA: IASP Press, 1994, 59-74.

Imedio EL. *Enfermera en Cuidados Paliativos (The Nurse in Palliative Care)* [in Spanish]. Madrid: Editorial Médica Panamerica, 1998.

Johnson SH, ed. Symposium: Legal and Regulatory Issues in Pain Management. *J Law Med Ethics* 1998;26(4):265-352.

Levin ML, Berry JI, Leiter J. Management of pain in terminally ill patients: Physician reports of knowledge, attitudes, and behavior. *J Pain Symptom Management* 1998;15(1):27-40.

McCaffery M, Pasero C. *Pain: Clinical Manual,* 2nd ed. St. Louis: CV Mosby, 1999.

Portenoy RK, Bruera E. *Topics in Palliative Care,* vol. 1. Oxford, UK: Oxford University Press, 1997.

Rischer JB, Childress SB. Cancer pain management: Pilot implementation of the AHCPR guideline in Utah. *J Quality Improvement* 1996;22(10):683-700.

Special Section on Measuring Quality of Care at Life's End. *J Pain Symptom Management* 1999;17(2):73-124.

Symptom Management. In: Doyle D, Hanks GWC, MacDonald N, eds. *Oxford Textbook of Palliative Medicine.* Oxford, UK: Oxford University Press, 1998, pp. 247-774.

Weissman DE, Dahl JW, Beasley JW. The cancer pain role model program of the Wisconsin Cancer Pain Initiative. *J Pain Symptom Management* 1993;8(1): 29-35.

Wisconsin Cancer Pain Initiative. *Building an Institutional Commitment to Pain Management: The Mayday Resource Manual for Improvement.* Madison, WI: University of Wisconsin Board of Regents, 1996.

World Health Organization Programme on Cancer Pain Control. Relevant publications include:
Cancer Pain Relief and Palliative Care in Children. Geneva, Switzerland: World Health Organization, 1998.
Symptom Relief in Terminal Illness. Geneva, Switzerland: World Health Organization, July 1998.
Cancer Pain Relief, 2nd ed. Geneva, Switzerland: World Health Organization, 1996.
Cancer Pain Relief and Palliative Care. Geneva, Switzerland: World Health Organization, 1990.

Part Five

Promoting Meaning in the Lives of Patients with Advanced Dementia

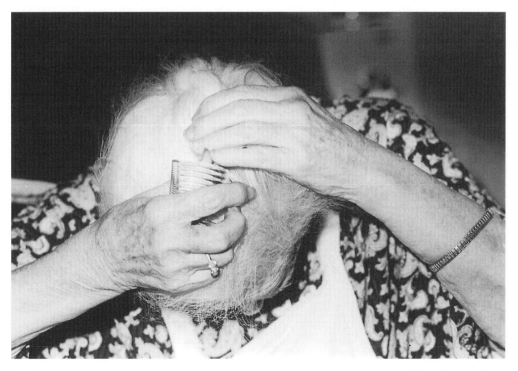

Only Connect: Promoting Meaning in the Lives of Patients with Advanced Dementia

ANNA L. ROMER, EdD

Education Development Center, Inc.
Newton, Massachusetts

Dementia is a condition that forces us to reconsider what span of time we are referring to when we use the term "end of life" and, even more importantly, what we mean by "life" and "meaning." How we define personhood changes when we consider a person suffering from dementia—a condition characterized by the progressive loss of memory and the cognitive abilities that anchor identity. Persons who suffer from Alzheimer's disease gradually lose their capacity to articulate their subjective experiences. Moreover, the close association of memory with making meaning has perhaps made it easy to assume that, with the loss of memory, meaning becomes irrelevant for people suffering from dementia.

Yet, the person suffering from dementia has much to teach others about what it is to be human and where one can find meaning. Our first memories are embodied: the touch of our mothers' warm skins; the taste of food; and the pleasurable feeling of moving our bodies through space. We internalize memories through our senses, such as when a particular bar of music releases a flood of feelings. The contributors to this part call on the power of the senses to evoke a response in persons with Alzheimer's disease. Their experiences suggest that stimulating sensory pathways can promote meaningful moments in the lives of people suffering from dementia when words no longer serve. We turn to E.M. Forster's injunction to "only connect" from his novel *Howards End*, as the red thread that weaves together these perspectives.[1] Each contributor attends carefully to ways to rejoin the person in the "patient" in the present moment, so that a connection is made that is meaningful to both people.

We open this part with a first-person narrative written by the husband in a couple married for more than 50 years about the new relationship he and his wife have created together in light of the changes brought about by her suffering from Alzheimer's disease (Separate and Yet Together: Living with a Spouse Suffering from Alzheimer's Disease, by Thomas Cassirer, see pages 145–150). We are intentionally asking our readers to begin this part about thoughtful current practice in dementia care with a story that brings the humanity of the person suffering from dementia and the personal experience of a close family member to center stage. In his unflinching commitment to join his wife where she is, Mr. Cassirer

> *. . . health care professionals and family members have a special responsibility to connect with these people who have lost the ability to make connections on their own. For this reason, quality end-of-life dementia care must include excellent physical care as well as attending to the psychological and spiritual needs of the individual.*

calls on all that he knows about her to find a space and activities that allow them to recreate a relationship that is meaningful and joyful to them both.

Defining and measuring quality of life has been a challenging focus of ongoing efforts in end-of-life care,[2] in part, because of its subjective nature. Bringing this concept to dementia care poses even tougher challenges because patients with mid-to-advanced-stage dementia cannot report back on their own subjective experiences.[3] Recently, researchers and clinicians have given greater attention to understanding the person of the patient and ways of promoting quality of life[4-6] and excellent palliative care for patients who suffer from Alzheimer's disease and related dementias.[7] Ladislav Volicer, MD, PhD, and Lisa Bloom-Charette, PhD, have edited a recently published book on this topic, entitled: *Enhancing Quality of Life in Advanced Dementia*, in which they lay out a conceptual model for defining quality of life and then proffer examples of innovative practice that focus on ways of increasing positive behaviors, rather than on managing or decreasing problematic behavior.[8]

In this part, we include two interviews with clinician–researchers working at the Edith Nourse Rogers Memorial Veterans Administration Hospital in Bedford, Massachusetts. The first interview focuses on the innovative conceptual work and research of Ladislav Volicer, MD, PhD, and Ann Hurley, RN, DNSc, FAAN, CNA. This physician–nurse researcher team discuss the ways in which their work and the field have evolved in recent years. Dr. Volicer speaks about his new model for understanding quality of life for patients suffering from dementia and Dr. Hurley discusses the particular contributions and considerations of nurses in providing end-of-life care for persons with dementia.

The second interview highlights the Bright Eyes program created by Scott A. Trudeau, MA, OTR/L, an occupational therapist who serves as clinical director for rehabilitation at the Edith Nourse Rogers Veterans Administration Hospital. Bright Eyes is a sensory stimulation program he designed based on Carol Bowlby's sensory stimulation hierarchy.[9] Mr. Trudeau has reported on the results of his research about the effectiveness of this intervention in Volicer and Bloom-Charette's new book.[10] In this part of *Innovations*, he describes the evolution and implementation of this program aimed at engaging persons with advanced Alzheimer's disease, including the ways his own thinking has been changed by this work.

In the International Perspectives section, we interview Mary T. Marshall, a professor at the Dementia Services Development Centre (DSDC) at the University of Stirling in Scotland about her work. An additional resource for information on international activity in dementia care can be found at the websites of the DSDC and of EACH (the European Alzheimer Clearing House), financed by the European

Community. These sites and others are provided in the Resources and Tools section in Appendix A.

We do not wish to underestimate the devastating effects of Alzheimer's disease and related dementias on all aspects of the patient's life, as well as on that of immediate family members. It is, in fact, against the backdrop of the enormous losses inflicted by dementia on patients and their families that the momentary victories these contributors describe become meaningful. Caregivers can still make a difference in the lives of patients who suffer from dementia. In fact, health care professionals and family members have a special responsibility to connect with these people who have lost the ability to make connections on their own. For this reason, quality end-of-life dementia care must include excellent physical care as well as attending to the psychological and spiritual needs of the individual. The creative efforts of our contributors begin to flesh out some concrete ways of doing that.

REFERENCES

1. Forster EM. *Howards End.* New York: Random House, 1921.
2. Volicer L, Bloom-Charette L. Assessment of quality of life in advanced dementia. In: L Volicer L, Bloom-Charette L, eds. *Enhancing the Quality of Life in Advanced Dementia*. Philadelphia: Taylor & Francis, 1999, pp. 3–20.
3. Rabins PV, Kasper JD. Measuring quality of life in dementia: Conceptual and practical issues. *Alzheimer's Disease & Associated Disorders* 1997;11:100–104.
4. Lawton MP. Assessing quality of life in Alzheimer's disease research. *Alzheimer's Disease & Associated Disorders* 1997;11:91–99.
5. Burgener SC. Quality of life in late-stage dementia. In: Volicer L, Hurley A, eds. *Hospice Care for Patients with Advanced Progressive Dementia*. New York: Springer Publishing, 1998, pp. 88–113.
6. Lyman K. *Day In, Day Out with Alzheimer's Care: Stress in Caregiving Relationships*. Philadelphia: Temple University Press, 1993.
7. Solomon MZ, Jennings B. Palliative care for Alzheimer patients: Implications for institutions, caregivers, and families. In: Volicer L, Hurley A, eds. *Hospice Care for Patients with Advanced Progressive Dementia*. New York: Springer Publishing, 1998, pp. 132–154.
8. Volicer L, Bloom-Charette L. *Enhancing Quality of Life in Advanced Dementia*. Philadelphia: Taylor & Francis, 1999.
9. Bowlby MC. *Therapeutic Activities with Persons Disabled by Alzheimer's Disease and Related Disorders*. Gaithersburg, MD: Aspen Publishers, 1993.
10. Trudeau SA. Bright Eyes: A structured sensory stimulation intervention. In: Volicer L, Bloom-Charette L, eds. *Enhancing the Quality of Life in Advanced Dementia*. Philadelphia: Taylor & Francis, 1999, pp. 93–106.

Personal Reflection

Separate and Yet Together: Living with a Spouse Suffering from Alzheimer's Disease

THOMAS CASSIRER

OUR LIFE BEFORE

Both of us, as children, were torn from our homes in Germany by the Nazi revolution and, via different itineraries, found ourselves by the age of 18 separated from our parents and living in North America. Some years later, we met in Montreal and eventually married on the slender funds offered by a graduate fellowship (hers) and an assistantship (mine) in the United States. We each launched careers in higher education, in which we introduced students to cultures outside the United States through the teaching of language and literature. Our marriage brought us a daughter, whose assistance was to be invaluable later in our lives during the crisis brought on by Alzheimer's disease.

In 1990 we both retired, triggering changes that gradually undermined our married life. We did not retire for the same reasons. My retirement was voluntary, brought on by the realization that it was time to end my career and explore on my own the potential of the Third Age of life. She, on the other hand, had no choice, because she belonged to the last generation who was subject to mandatory retirement. Consequently, she felt expelled from a career to which she had devoted 40 years, while I felt liberated from a bureaucratic lifestyle and free to do whatever I wanted. I believe this had a definite effect on the course of her Alzheimer's disease, and perhaps the inverse is also true—the early, unrecognized stages of Alzheimer's disease may have narrowed her range of responses to this new challenge. She experienced the loss of her position as a loss of support, almost as being thrust back into the predicament of her youth, when she had to find a "ladder" that would allow her to climb to the level of her intellectual capacity. But now in retirement there was no such ladder, and though she remained physically very vigorous she could not, at her age, repeat the climb of her youth. She felt herself diminished whereas I felt my life expanding now that I was freed from the limitations imposed by my job. Over the years, this difference in our orientations caused increasing conflict between us, while, at the same time, she became more and more dependent on me because of what I now recognize as the inroads of Alzheimer's disease.

Our life as a couple collapsed in the fiftieth year of our marriage. In the years since our retirement, I had become involved in ever more strenuous caregiving because she refused all medical intervention with the argument that she was in perfect health (which was true of her physical constitution) and that doctors made you sick in order to make money. In November 1997, I collapsed with severe pneumonia. Because she insisted on treating me herself at home, and the only friend to whom she might have turned for help happened to be out of town, I would probably not have survived if she had not gone to the post office to collect my mail. The woman behind the counter, who knew us both, suspected that my absence meant that something was wrong and notified her supervisor, who notified the police. The police found me semiconscious, but able to signal that I wanted to go to the hospital. They warded off an attack by my wife, who wanted to keep me home, and took both of us to the hospital. There, my wife was diagnosed as suffering from Alzheimer's disease. The hospital called our daughter, who flew in and took over her parents' lives. Our daughter discovered a newly opened assisted-living facility for Alzheimer's patients and was able to place her mother there, while I spent more than 3 weeks in the hospital before I began the slow mend back to health.

Our married life had disintegrated. It was out of the question for us to ever live together again. Now we had to build a new relationship. Each of us had to learn to lead a new life in a new location (I sold the house and moved into a condominium). From now on, we would live separately—but could we also be together?

THE NEW LIFE

What follows is a brief narrative of the trial-and-error problem-solving process through which we learned, over the course of about a year, how we could lead separate lives and yet also be together to the point where our relationship has become happier and more satisfying than it had been in the later years of our marriage. Or, to say the same in her words, "We used to yell a lot at each other and now we don't any more. How come?"

The word "we" in the preceding paragraph is deliberate because in her own way she has participated in this process and in many ways has set the conditions. Because she has consistently denied that she is suffering from any illness, she has refused all medication, even vitamins, and will not let herself be treated as a patient. When, after weeks of recuperation, I first visited her, she called out, "My Dad has come back!" Since then, she usually refers to me as "Dad" and to herself as my daughter. When I told her our daughter would be returning for a visit, she said, "And then you will have two daughters." This is when I started to learn her new language, which frequently expresses her emotions rather than her perception of external reality.

What was she telling me by identifying me as "Dad"? She wasn't confusing me with my father-in-law. She refers to him as "my father," or sometimes as "my other father." What I eventually understood was that by calling me "Dad" she was acknowledging her dependence on me, a radical change from the independent, self-directed professional woman who had been my partner for so many years. She also told me clearly that she relied on me to orient her so she would not get lost and said that I had to act as her memory since hers was no longer so good. As

"Dad" of this Alzheimer "child" in her upper 70s, I had to see to it that she was protected from the world at large in which she could no longer orient herself. It was up to me to find a world "her size" in which we could be together and she could feel at home and safe. But that presented quite a problem: How could I provide such a home when living with her had proved quite literally life-threatening for me? The assisted-living residence provided for her need to be safe and taken care of, but it did not offer us a space that was ours and in which we could create a home for ourselves.

> *Moreover, she had not merely lost her home; the crisis had also reduced to a shadowy memory the substance of her 40 years as a teacher and scholar. What remained were the two vital resources, walking and music, that have propelled her since adolescence and that brought us together in 1945, well before it became evident that she was headed for the academic career she has now forgotten.*

Moreover, she had not merely lost her home; the crisis had also reduced to a shadowy memory the substance of her 40 years as a teacher and scholar. What remained were the two vital resources, walking and music, that have propelled her since adolescence and that brought us together in 1945, well before it became evident that she was headed for the academic career she has now forgotten. Any space that might be "ours," that could hold us together even while we lived separately, had to be a space that allowed her access to these two vital resources. But what did she mean by "walking" and "music"? Everyone walks, and almost everyone appreciates some form of music, but that was not what she meant.

Walking gave expression to the freedom of her body as it relied on its inherent strength and perfect functioning to carry her wherever she wished to go. Her walking was at its high point during our annual summer vacations in the Swiss and Austrian Alps, when we used our bodies to the fullest, hiking day after day from one mountain shelter to the next. On these occasions she used to say, "When I am above 2000 meters, I could walk to the end of the world." Not being as good a walker as she, I was often secretly afraid that one day she might do just that. Walking energized her entire body and her mind as well. She much preferred to talk with friends while walking, rather than sitting down. Walking by herself—and, in later years driving—was her favorite way of relieving tension. In her present condition she still had her physical energy, but she had lost her sense of orientation and no longer felt free to walk by herself. Could I help her regain that sense of freedom?

For the meaning of "music," she also returned to her youth. She rejected the musical activity at the assisted-living residence because it consisted mainly of American popular music from the youth of the great majority of residents who grew up in New England during the 1930s and 1940s. In her mind, she returned to the classical music to which she had been introduced at the conservatory during her adolescence in Germany. Above all, she returned to Johann Sebastian Bach, whose music she discovered largely on her own and which has inspired her throughout her entire life.

This needs some explanation: She was sent to the conservatory on the recommendation of her teachers. Her father was proud to have such a gifted child, but would not let her play when he was home because he did not care for music. Her mother, a native Viennese who felt exiled in "provincial" Germany, welcomed the opportunity to have her daughter play tunes from the Viennese operettas of her youth, but did not want to hear music that was too serious. Outside the apartment, in the streets of Nazi Germany, the air resounded with the songs and military music of the Nazi movement. In that atmosphere of confusion and hostility she discovered in the music of Johann Sebastian Bach a world of order and beauty. It became her lifetime inspiration and, in a sense, her shield against the outside world.

When she was a girl, this situation was rendered even more difficult by the fact that, in order to hear Bach, she had to go into Protestant churches. But she was brought up a Catholic and, at that time, it was a sin for a Catholic girl to go to a Protestant place of worship. It took her mother's reassurance to convince her that she did not need to confess this "sin."

Now she again felt imprisoned, as she used to feel in Nazi Germany; to the point that during the first difficult months in assisted living, she sometimes referred to the personnel as "jailers," even though the facility offers as much freedom as is compatible with the need to keep the residents from wandering. When she managed to escape (she can move with amazing speed) and was brought back by the police, she described this to me as an attack by a group of storm troopers. She again turned to the music of Bach to sustain her, which helped her get over periods of depression, especially when the more rhythmic compositions set her off into energetic dancing. However, I did not understand the full meaning of "music" to her until I took her, on a Sunday afternoon in October 1998, to a performance of two Bach cantatas on the town green. She was in constant motion in her seat as the music flowed through her body; she was moved emotionally as well as physically, as I have seldom seen her, both by the performance and by the feeling of oneness with the very appreciative audience. Suddenly, I became aware of something I should have realized long ago: This music put her in touch with a harmonious social order and lifted her above the many conflicts in her life. Six months later, she was still asking me for another such performance on "the Green" (she does not remember the name of the town).

> *I have built up a routine that is now so familiar to her that it would be more appropriate to call these occasions our "homings" rather than our "outings."*

Out of all these elements I had to construct a space that was "ours," where we could be together, as one is in a home, but not confined as one is in a house. I eventually found the space at the Quabbin, a 22-mile-long reservoir that supplies much of Boston's water. It is surrounded by densely forested hills and at its southern end is open to the public, with a network of trails for hiking and a lookout tower on the highest hill from which one can view the entire vast space of water and forest.

We have been going regularly to the Quabbin for more than eight months now. During that period, I have built up a routine that is now so familiar to her that it would be more appropriate to call these occasions our "homings" rather than our "outings."

Sunday is the day when classical music is most likely to be performed in the afternoon. (I cannot take her to an evening concert because it frightens her when we drive in the dark.) That may have been the superficial reason why I chose Sunday as our regular day but, after a while, I came to realize that it had become our day of communion—not with any particular faith or congregation, but a day of communion with the universe, with the sky, the water and woods that rise from the shore and reach up toward the horizon; a day when, in warmer weather, we can walk barefoot in the grass and find a quiet spot on a meadow or in the woods where we can rest or even snooze. It is a day of solitude because we often are the only people walking the trails, yet also a day when she can mingle with the families out for a stroll and enjoy the feeling of being in a "normal" social setting with many children and teenagers—and can do so without the fear that she might run into an acquaintance or friend from former times who might greet her and unintentionally remind her that she had forgotten those who still remembered her.

Here again it was she who made me aware of the deeper meaning of the Quabbin, as she drew my attention to the sky and the landscape in which no human habitation could be seen. She got to know the trails and could tell me which trail she wanted to take. She felt particularly drawn to the lookout tower on the highest hill, because from there she could "see the whole world." This was also the time when I turned the car into a "moving home." While sitting in the car and looking out over the reservoir, we would have a picnic lunch consisting primarily of the kind of bread she liked and "Deutschmacher" frankfurters that really taste like German "wurst." The lunch was consumed to the accompaniment of a cassette of music by Bach and she got many a laugh out of this German combination of sausage and Bach.

Through comedy of this type and by introducing "interesting questions" into our conversation, I would see to it that she also got some "mental exercise." I recall one day when I used her father's expressions which were somewhat off-color and very funny—the type he would use over beer with his business colleagues. I started a discussion on the difference between German and American joking. She got so interested that she urged me to look for literature on the subject and said she would love to help me write this up. (The next week, she had of course forgotten all about this.) Recently, she discovered the memorial stone to the chief engineer who directed the building of the Quabbin; she gave me, in a somewhat confused way, a feminist critique of this memorial, and, last Sunday, she said she needed to look at this memorial again and see this man who took all the credit for the Quabbin.

On days when there is no suitable concert, we usually wind up driving to a nearby town for a visit to an Italian café. She does not drink coffee and is not particularly interested in sweet pastries, but the café represents for her the epitome of urban life, especially on the days when we also have time to stroll along Main Street, with its many shops. After such a Sunday, she usually concludes, "This is the best yet," and is quite ready to return to the assisted-living residence, as long as I assure her that I will come again soon.

One final remark on these "homings" and the new relationship we have developed. While her face lights up immediately when I show up at the assisted-living residence and she is always very happy and affectionate, she wavers in her identification of exactly who I am. At times I am one of a group of "Thomases," and she tells me about another Thomas who visited her the previous week. At other times, when we arrive back at the residence, she acts as though we had been out on a very enjoyable date, hopes that I will come again soon to take her out, reminds me of her name, and adds, "But I don't know your name." It is evident that she feels there are at least two of me—the one who is with her and the other who is out somewhere, who is leading a life that she cannot imagine but who is likely to turn up at some other time. Again she is right, though her language is not what we who are "on the outside" consider normal, because I do lead two lives, one together with her on Sundays, and the other on my own in another world, yet, with her tucked away in my mind just as the "other Thomases" are tucked away in her mind.

SOME FINAL COMMENTS

First, a comment on the economic context that has allowed us to find a solution to our problem. We very probably could not afford this life if we had not married in 1948 with the explicit understanding that we would both have professional careers in order to insure us against unforeseen emergencies and give us freedom to lead the life we wanted. In the setting of that time, with its conventions that were so different from today's American life, our decision was viewed as contrary to what an American marriage should be. My wife was frequently penalized for her refusal to conform. But if we had done things differently, where would we be today? My hope is that for younger generations this solution of "separate, yet together" will be available to more couples because they will arrive at our age with the earnings of two individuals.

My other comment concerns the responsibilities of the "parent" of a spouse suffering from Alzheimer's. When I brought up my daughter, I was familiar with the adult world and therefore qualified to guide her toward her life as an adult. But my wife and I belong to the same generation. How can I be sure that as "Dad" I give her the right guidance toward a future that is as unknown to me as it is to her? I don't have a ready answer, and probably never will, but I am confident that a sequence of happy Sundays will strengthen her for whatever is in store, just as it strengthens both of us right now. I also believe that the weekly communion with the basic elements of our existence—the water, the earth, the vegetation nourished by water and earth, and the sky that opens our eyes to the universe—that all this orients us toward what transcends our individual lives. And, finally, I believe that the strong rhythm of Johann Sebastian Bach, which she has always identified as the rhythm of a "walking man," will keep us in touch with the human spirit, even when words can no longer do so.

In this section, we feature the work of three clinician-researchers, all based at the Geriatric Research and Education Clinical Center at the Edith Nourse Rogers Veterans Administration Hospital in Bedford, Massachusetts. This setting is the home of the Dementia Special Care Unit, a 100-bed inpatient unit, as well as an outpatient program, and an adult day care center for US veterans with dementia (the Veterans' Center). The Veterans Administration Health Care System, which is funded by the U.S. government and provides care for a large number of older patients, has taken advantage of the particular features of its centralized funding as well as its mandate to care for this aging population to become a leader in dementia care. In the following interview, Ladislav Volicer, MD, PhD, and Ann Hurley, RN, DNSc, FAAN, CNA, describe their research and its implications for practice. In the second interview, Scott A. Trudeau, MA, OTR/L, outlines the sensory stimulation program he designed, entitled Bright Eyes.

Caring for Patients with Advanced Dementia: Implications of Innovative Research for Practice

An Interview with ANN HURLEY, RN DNSc, FAAN, CNA,
and LADISLAV VOLICER, MD, PhD

*Edith Nourse Veterans Administration Hospital
New Bedford, Massachusetts*

Ladislav Volicer, MD, PhD, and Ann Hurley, RN, DNSc, FAAN, CNA, have conducted conceptually innovative research for more than 10 years on many specific elements of the care of patients with advanced dementia. This physician–nurse team has changed the way we think about dementia and how to provide quality palliative care for this group of patients, who have not been well served in this domain. Wide dissemination and implementation of their findings into clinical practice, however, have lagged. In this interview with Anna L. Romer, EdD, Drs. Volicer and Hurley explore the barriers to adoption of the principles that have emerged from their research and clinical experience. In addition, they talk about their current work, including Dr. Volicer's new model for quality of life and Dr. Hurley's insights about the importance of understanding the patient's experience as an entry point to providing quality care. They review the interdisciplinary process of meeting with families to determine goals and levels of care for patients with advanced demen-

tia, which they initiated at the Dementia Special Care Unit several years ago, and describe how the entire field of palliative care for dementia has evolved in recent years.

AN EVOLVING RESEARCH AGENDA AND A NEW DEFINITION OF QUALITY OF LIFE

Anna L. Romer: *How has your research focus evolved?*

Ladislav Volicer: The trajectory of our work seems to follow our evolving understanding of what makes up quality of life for patients with moderate-to-severe dementia. If you look at the model of quality of life that Lisa Bloom-Charette [PhD] and I describe in our new book you'll see that we define quality of life as made up of three main areas: medical symptoms; psychiatric symptoms; and the domain of meaningful activities.[1] We have a graphic with three intersecting circles, each representing one of these domains. The interfaces of each overlapping circle are also important. We define the interaction of medical symptoms and psychiatric symptoms as the domain of *comfort*; we define the interaction of psychiatric/ behavioral issues and meaningful activities as *mood* with the potential for depression; finally, our definition of the interaction of meaningful activities and medical symptoms involves the domain of *mobility*.

In our earliest research, we concentrated on medical concerns first. That early research investigated the treatment of infections, as well as eating difficulties and how to manage them, and we wrote a number of papers that made it clear that the most intrusive medical intervention might not always be appropriate in terms of patients' best interests and comfort.[2-4] Our second area of research focus has been psychiatric problems and understanding the behavior of patients with dementia. We are now pursuing this domain quite actively. The overlapping area of comfort has also been a major focus of ours from the beginning. Ann and other colleagues developed an objective scale for measuring discomfort in noncommunicative patients and evaluated it back in 1992.[5] We are continuing to pursue medical issues, for example, nutritional issues—determining optimal weight in Alzheimer's patients. When these patients lose their ability to ambulate, they lose muscle, and so their ideal body weight tables do not apply. To keep patients at a weight recommended for otherwise healthy adults would mean replacing the muscle with the fat, which is not in the patient's best interest.

However, the emphasis of our work is shifting from the medical to psychiatric and behavioral problems and, from there, to the issue of appropriate meaningful activities, which is where we are going and where we are still trying to improve our practice here at the Dementia Special Care Unit.

Ann Hurley: What I'm working on right now is a good example of the shift that Ladi is referring to. Dr. Ellen Mahoney from Boston College and I are leading a team investigating "resistiveness" to care. I find the following analogy helpful: Pain management is to cancer as behavioral symptom management—i.e., managing some of the problematic behaviors—is to dementia. There are the various stages of dementia and there are some behavioral problems that become intense during particular stages but, as the person gets more ill, he or she no longer has the physical capacity to mount some of those responses.

For instance, not being able to eat might happen at a very late stage, whereas some of the other "disruptive" problems might happen in the moderate stage of dementia. One of the foci of the program here, in addition to providing palliative care, is providing good quality care that includes managing the patient's aversive symptoms, just as managing pain is very important to cancer patients.

UNDERSTANDING THE PATIENT'S PERSPECTIVE CHANGES THE RESPONSE TO "PROBLEMATIC BEHAVIOR"

AH: One of the issues is that patients don't always understand what's happening to them. For instance, if I were to bathe a person who couldn't understand what I was doing, and I just brought him or her into a tub room that was cold and used a hydraulic lift to plunge that person into cold water, that would be a very frightening situation. If we just invade a person's territory, tear off his or her clothes, and march in with a wet face cloth, then the person will want to protect him or herself and, if I still persist, the person would want to ward me off and then might end up hitting me. One of the things you want to do is to avoid those situations you know are frightening. We have done several studies in which we analyzed videotapes of these caregiving encounters. If you don't look at the whole scene on the videotape you might think some of those problematic behaviors come out of the blue, but very often there is a precipitant within the caregiving encounter. So, first we have developed a scale to measure resistance to care, and second we've looked at several interventions during bathing to decrease resistiveness to care. My agenda this summer is working with Dr. Mahoney, who's the project director for this grant, to complete the analyses.

ALR: *How do you measure resistiveness?*

AH: Resistiveness has several components. It's got intensity, frequency, and numbers of resistive behaviors, and let's say, collectively, these components add up to the severity of the resistiveness. If you can intervene with any of those—if you can decrease the number of resistive behaviors or how long they persist and how strong they are—then you can make a difference in terms of resistiveness. Our resistiveness-to-care scale is a 13-item form that gets rated in terms of presence, duration, and intensity during the rating period.[6]

LV: I would like to add to that. The goal is really to try to prevent resistiveness. That's what the tapes are used for, to look at the antecedent model and antecedent signs and to find out how we can prevent the escalation of uncooperative behavior into resistiveness.

AH: One issue that many professionals find distressing is almost a "blame-the-victim" phenomenon. Many of the problematic behaviors that patients suffering from dementia engage in are distressing to staff. It's distressing when someone hits you, it's distressing to other patients when they hear someone hollering, and it's distressing to families and visitors, too. And so sometimes the incentive for addressing these problems is to decrease the burden on caregivers. My reaction is, "Let's step back! This person with dementia must be suffering so much internally if that's the external symptomatology." So one of my major interests is to focus on that person's internal experience. If a patient is acting in a way that's troublesome, get to the root of the problem.

ALR: *Is the point of view and approach you've just described prevalent in the literature and in clinical practice?*

AH: No, it's not as widely practiced as it should be. A lot of the literature still points to distressing behaviors, disruptive behaviors, and obstreperous behaviors. Even the labeling of some of the instruments that are used to assess those behaviors have a blame-the-victim cast to them. For example, one tool has the acronym COBRA (the Caretaker Obstreperous Behavior Rating Assessment).[7] The cobra is a snake. To label a tool for measuring behavior by the name of COBRA is distasteful to me.

LV: This connects to Ann's approach to the issue of resistiveness and why Ann is so interested in trying to change the mindset of people who call Alzheimer patients "aggressive" or "assaultive." If you really look at it, they are not assaultive or aggressive when you leave them alone. They just get upset if somebody is touching them—somebody is trying to do something with them and they don't understand what's going on. It's distressing to patients. So, it's not really that they are themselves assaultive or aggressive, it's really just because of the confusion. That's why we call it "resistiveness" and try to get away from this assaultive, aggressive, obstreperous behavior type of terminology.

AH: I'd like to get away from blaming the victim, to try to understand how painful, how uncomfortable, how distressing and disturbing someone must feel internally if he or she is acting that way. Ladi elaborated on resistiveness to care, that we look at it within the behavioral model of ABC—which refers to Antecedent, Behavior, Consequences. Now, when we are trying to understand resistive behavior, we look for the antecedents. For instance, when Ladi was doing a nursing-home consultation, he was consulted about a patient who really acted out during bathing. Well, it turned out that the person had metastatic cancer with pathological bone fractures for which she was not receiving proper analgesia!

There's another cluster of behaviors that draw less attention and is related to persons who are apathetic, withdraw into themselves, don't interact with the environment, and are not troublesome. These people don't get the attention that they need, which you can understand. If there are few staff members and one patient is hollering and another is withdrawn, who's going to get the attention? Not the poor persons sitting all by themselves, doing nothing. It's up to us to be proactive, to provide meaningful activities and joy and pleasure for those persons that don't demand it of us.

A CULTURAL SHIFT IN APPROACH TO CARE

ALR: *Let's look beyond your work to the larger culture of care. What's changed over the past 10 years or so? Has there been a shift?*

LV: There is certainly a shift away from providing aggressive interventions for Alzheimer's patients; for instance, the use of tube feeding for patients with advanced dementia has decreased very, very markedly in the past years. It's also recognized that it's not always appropriate to transfer patients from nursing homes to acute-care settings for treatment of infection and so on. There are a lot of people who are trying to treat these infections in the nursing homes to avoid the transfer.

ALR: *Why is it so important not to transfer patients with dementia to acute-care settings?*

LV: The acute-care setting is not very good for patients with dementia. The staff there don't know how to handle these patients. It's not a safe setting; they usually have to be restrained in bed because they would remove their IVs. They would wander around and might be unsafe in that environment, so, it's a very distressing experience for them. Very often these patients develop pressure sores; they develop contractures; their nutritional status gets worse because, again, the acute-care staff doesn't know how to feed them and might not have time to feed them appropriately; and so on. So, as much as that can be avoided, it's certainly in the best interest of the patient not to be moved. There is actually a study that indicates that acute survival is the same in the hospital and nursing home, and long-term survival is actually better in patients who are treated in a nursing home than those who are transferred to a hospital.[8]

AH: Beyond the potential iatrogenesis, there is also the factor of the long-term care staff knowing the patient. They know patients' nuances, what they like, what they dislike, and sometimes they know the patients' immediate needs better than their loved ones do, which is very sad for the wives who see this phenomenon between a veteran and the staff. The staff spends more hours with the veteran than the spouse does, and some of the veterans respond better to the staff than they do to the spouse. Patients start to forget who they are and who their loved ones are. Yet these same patients become quasi-secure in this long-term care environment where they know the staff and the routines are familiar. To move a patient with dementia away from this familiar environment to someplace new is a problem.

NURSES' ROLE IN ADVANCE CARE PLANNING

AH: One of the projects that we had done shortly after I came on board is looking at the role of the nurse in what we then called advance care planning, or advance proxy planning. These are discussions that go on in the absence of written advance care planning documents, or if existing documents need more elaboration for patients with severe dementia who are near the end of their lives.

The team develops a plan and elicits preferences from the family about what the family wants to have done in terms of providing comfort care or palliative care as the disease marches on and predictable complications occur. The family, in concert with the caregiving team, makes these decisions on behalf of the veteran. This project was one of the first efforts to bring hospice/palliative-care services to patients with advanced dementia.[9-10]

The process of opening a discussion with family members about the treatment of disease symptoms in patients suffering from an advanced stage of dementia came out of our belief that we should be changing the paradigm of care at this point from *high-tech* to *high-touch* care.[11] Aggressive medical interventions at this stage may or may not extend a patient's life and often cause discomfort as well as increasing the likelihood of iatrogenic complications. Given our understanding of the clinical and ethical issues for these patients' care, we were striving to create a system that made patient comfort the highest priority and attended to patient and family values.

Within this model of care, five levels of care were developed. Level One involves patients receiving aggressive diagnostic workups, treatment of coexisting medical conditions, and transfer to acute-care units if necessary. This level includes using CPR in the event of cardiac arrest and tube feeding if normal food intake is not possible. Each subsequent level involves implementing less aggressive/intrusive care. Patients in Level Two are assigned DNR status [Do Not Resuscitate], but otherwise receive the same care as Level One. Level Three involves DNR and no acute care unit transfer for medical management of intercurrent life-threatening illness. Level Four involves all the previous restrictions, and no workup or antibiotic treatment for life-threatening infections. Antipyretics and analgesics are used for patient comfort. These have been shown to be equally effective and less invasive for patients. Level Five includes supportive care as defined by the fourth level, but eliminates tube feeding by nasogastric tube or gastrostomy when normal food intake is not possible. Each level of care is not only defined by what medical interventions are *not* applied, but by intensive care nursing interventions that *are* applied. For example, nurses offer many comfort measures to manage fever symptoms for patients.

This process of negotiating care levels begins with the team of nurses who provide the care that the veteran receives 24 hours a day, seven days a week, getting together with the unit physician to come to consensus on what to recommend as the level of care to the family member at the family conference. The providers have all this knowledge, and we believe that it would be stressful and even irresponsible to say to the family member, "Here's a blank piece of paper, we're not going to give you our recommendations at all, this is what you can do." Instead, the nurses get together with the ward physician, talk about the status of the person, and come up with a recommendation they believe is in the patient's best interest. It's a recommendation for the family to consider, not necessarily accept.

The family conference is an essential part of this process. The family member(s), with the assistance of the physician, the nurse, the social worker, the chaplain, and whomever the family wants to bring, really grapples with the problems that are facing their loved one now. What does the immediate future look like? What decisions does the surrogate decision maker need to make in advance about the care that the veteran should receive?

When the program first began, there wasn't as much agreement between the nurse's recommendations and what the family ultimately decided as there is now. This is something that Ladi and I have talked about. My perspective is that the nurse cannot help but consider the patient in the whole-family context. Now Ladi will keep bringing the staff back to say: "What do you think is best for the veteran?" The team makes a recommendation in terms of the whole family, but the family member bears responsibility for making this decision, which can be very difficult to do.

UNDERSTANDING IMPLICATIONS OF TREATMENT CHOICES

AH: In fact, we have observed that families sometimes believe that aggressive treatments have more power than they really do, i.e., a greater likelihood of "success" in overcoming the natural course of the disease than they really do. Ellen Robinson, RN, PhD, did her dissertation on the experience of the family member who makes an advance directive and advance care plan, and then actually lives through the implementation of that plan. Ellen interviewed some of the wives, and one of the stories she told me about a veteran's wife talking about DNR was particularly poignant. This particular veteran did not need to be resuscitated because he didn't have an event in which his heart stopped or his breathing stopped. But, as she considered this decision in the abstract, she would say, "I put it on, and I took it off, and I put it on, then I took it off." This struggle to make what seemed to be a life-and-death decision was occurring in the absence of an understanding of the very low likelihood of CPR being effective in an unwitnessed arrest in a demented person who is severely enough demented to require long-term care. So, she was agonizing about a theoretical possibility, i.e., the possibility of bringing him back to life, which really wasn't grounded in reality. That's

One more thing I'd like to emphasize is that this is a process, and that some people worship at the shrine of the legally executed advance directive. Some doctors do that so they can wipe their hands and go away, they don't bother to talk with the family again. But this is an ongoing process. Communication and trust-building are so important throughout.

what I mean when I say that people often invest choices regarding treatment with more power than studies of the consequences of those interventions show to be true.

One more thing I'd like to emphasize is that this is a process, and that some people worship at the shrine of the legally executed advance directive. Some doctors do that so they can wipe their hands and go away, they don't bother to talk with the family again. But this is an ongoing process. Communication and trust-building are so important throughout.

CURRENT RESEARCH

ALR: *What are you working on right now?*

LV: We are finishing a study in which we surveyed family members of recently deceased patients with Alzheimer's disease about the survivors' caregiving experiences. The purpose of this study was to develop recommendations for policy changes that would remove some of the barriers interfering with appropriate end-of-life care for patients suffering from Alzheimer's. Some of the barriers which we identified were lack of support for home care and day care and, of course, the requirement for a 6-month survival prognosis to be eligible for hospice care.

CHANGING PRACTICE BASED ON THE QUALITY-OF-LIFE MODEL

ALR: *How does your new model for defining quality of life for patients with advanced dementia translate into changes in practice?*

LV: In the three-circle model I described earlier, what's important are the medical issues, psychiatric issues and behavior, and meaningful activity. Only when patient needs in all of these domains are met can we talk about providing high quality of life for the patients.

Enhancing Mobility

LV: The interface between meaningful activities and medical issues is *mobility*, which is very important because movement, specifically walking, provides an outlet for physical energy and some meaningful activity for people with dementia. Just walking around is very useful. It helps them do something that they like. So it's very important to try to preserve mobility as long as possible and it's important for long-term care institutions to create safe spaces for patients to walk in without getting lost.

At the same time, lack of mobility has medical consequences. When patients are unable to ambulate any more, they have higher incidence of pneumonia, urinary tract infections, and, of course, pressure sores.

AH: I'll just comment on one more thing on mobility. Dr. Robinson, who interviewed the wives relative to living through their decisions, found that one of the concepts that came through loud and clear was the meaning of loss of mobility to the wives. As the disease progresses and the patient gets worse—when it ratchets down to that someone can't walk—that's just a milestone for them. So, what we can do to use assistive devices to maintain mobility, such as the "merrywalker," is very important. The merrywalker is a device similar to the walkers children sometimes use before they can walk independently. The patient can lean on the frame for balance, get mobility assistance from the wheels, and sit back on a sling if tired without risk of falling and hurting him or herself.

ALR: *Are devices like the merrywalker commonly available in less-privileged long-term care settings than the Geriatric Research and Education Clinical Center?*

LV: Yes. There are several models, actually, of these care devices. Some of them are better than others. Some of them are awfully big and made out of plastic tubes and so on. But it depends on the setting. If you have a lot of space, probably it doesn't make that much difference. But they are available, although not everyone uses them.

Enhancing Comfort

The interaction between the medical and psychiatric issues leads to questions of comfort, which we already discussed. That's very important, and it points to the importance of trying to provide appropriate medical care rather than inappropriate, aggressive medical care.

Overly aggressive medical care for patients in late stages of dementia just increases the discomfort of the patient without any benefit to the patient. Because, as we showed, in advanced dementia, antibiotic treatment, which usually requires aggressive interventions as well, is not really beneficial. The use of antibiotics does not increase comfort. We found, using the scale that Ann designed, that you can keep patients as comfortable by using antipyretics and analgesics as if you gave them antibiotics.

Treating Depression

The third interface is between the meaningful activities and the psychiatric symptoms, and that brings up the issue of mood—with possible depression, which is very common in patients with Alzheimer's. Yet, depression is often underdiagnosed and undertreated because psychiatrists sometimes look for more verbal expressions and more verbal symptoms, which the patients with dementia are unable to provide because of their speech difficulties. So, you really have to look more at nonverbal symptoms of depression—facial expressions, moods, food intakes, sleep, and things like that. Often, antidepressant treatment improves behavioral symptoms very much, allowing the patient to participate in activities and therefore improve his or her quality of life.

ALR: *How many of the patients on your inpatient unit are on antidepressants combined with structured activities to treat depression?*

LV: Probably half of our patients are on antidepressants.

BARRIERS TO IMPLEMENTATION

ALR: *You've described your treatment philosophy, which is supported by scientific data, yet, this approach to dementia care is not generally adopted in most nursing homes. Why is it so hard to implement these understandings? What are the barriers?*

AH: I wish I knew. That's a study on its own. A nurse colleague once said, "Much as I love to do research, a part of me thinks you should call a moratorium on doing new research until we get people to use what we already know." I don't have the answer, but we do have to promote research utilization to promote evidence-based care.

LV: One of the barriers to implementation is existing policies. Some current policies are inappropriate or actually misguided, for instance, the issue of hospice and the requirement of a prognosis of less than six-month survival. The prognosis for six-month survival is very, very difficult to determine in patients with Alzheimer's because it's very difficult to predict how long they will live. It's such an unpredictable disease—even patients in very, very late stages of dementia sometimes live for years because they don't develop infections, which are the most common cause of death in this condition. So, the requirement of six month's prognosis eliminates or excludes a lot of patients who would be very appropriate for a palliative approach to care.

Education is clearly a problem, especially in nursing homes, where the staff turnover is so rapid. According to our experience, it takes up to a year for people who are relatively new to this kind of setting to learn to deal with this patient population and to become fully functional and fully aware. So, if you have a 100-percent turnover rate of nursing assistants in nursing homes, it's very difficult to have staff who really know how to deal with individuals suffering from dementia. This lack of staff continuity leads to low-quality care.

Lack of advance care planning among this population is another problem. Patients and families don't plan ahead of time. That's one of the biggest issues, too.

We are trying to push proxy planning, which Ann described, and the involvement of the nursing staff such that you make the decision ahead of a crisis situation, in terms of the treatment limitations, resuscitation, transfer to an acute care setting, use of antibiotics, and things like that.

ALR: *When would it be responsible to transfer a patient with dementia to a hospital?*

LV: It certainly would be important for an issue of comfort. For instance, if someone who was still walking breaks a hip and that hip can be repaired, fixing the hip certainly would require transfer to a hospital.

ALR: *What other kinds of policies would you like to see in long-term care settings that have many patients with dementia, in terms of improving practice?*

LV: Eliminating tube feeding and just continuing feeding by natural means, by changing diet and using correct nursing strategies.

AH: When we talk at other VAs and in the community, people say, "Well, all right, you can feed by natural means, but you must have an army of people in your GRECC unit!" Surprise, surprise, we are staffed with fewer people than there are in the community in terms of the ratio of providers to veterans. Seeing is believing, so we invited people to come on up to the GRECC and see what the staff here does even with limited numbers of people. Nursing staff alter the consistency of the food and use strategies to get around eating difficulties. Persons with Alzheimer's disease can do a number of things to refuse food. Are they pouching it, i.e., keeping the food in their cheeks? Do they kiss the spoon? We developed a videotape so that people could see our approaches to dealing with these challenges without having to come to Bedford. You need to provide instruction if you want others to implement the findings of your research or to try something new, like using natural feeding techniques instead of tube feeding.

LV: I'm not sure I agree with Ann about the staffing ratios, actually. But I think the staffing is similar. I wouldn't say that our staffing is worse than what's on the outside.

ALR: *But it sounds as though you have lower staff turnover and that the staff here have learned these somewhat complex routines for how to deal with people refusing food so that patients can continue to be fed naturally.*

> *That's the most important—the staff education and also staff supervision. I think it's important to provide supervision with RNs and LPNs over the nursing assistants. Unless you have that very careful supervision, there is no way to know if good care is actually provided.*

LV: That's the most important—the staff education and also staff supervision. I think it's important to provide supervision with RNs and LPNs over the nursing assistants. Unless you have that very careful supervision, there is no way to know if good care is actually provided.

AH: When the Alzheimer's Association revised the pamphlet "Key Elements of Dementia Care," we were asked to do the chapter on staffing, and we wouldn't commit to a number. Everyone wants the ideal staff–patient ratio—the number, the number!—so they can show a piece of paper to somebody.

ALR: *Why wouldn't you commit to a number?*

AH: Because things are so variable that one nursing assistant doesn't equal another nursing assistant. For instance, there are some nursing assistants at the Bedford VA who are superb. They have been on the units for years and years, just love the patients, and it shows, whereas, in some community nursing homes, the staff member might be a poorly paid minimum-wage earner, a mother with a delinquent payer of child support who is trying to keep body and soul together and doesn't have the training or the understanding, and had to take the job because there was no other job available. It's hard to get people for some of those positions. Five unmotivated or overwhelmed-by-life nursing assistants don't equal one superb nursing assistant.

ALR: *Any parting thoughts?*

LV: Especially when we talk about end-of-life care, it is important to remember that even patients with very advanced dementia are still aware of the environment and still require comfort measures. These people still require stimulation, meaningful activity, or meaningful environmental stimulation. There are some people who claim that patients with advanced dementia get into a persistent vegetative state, but I strongly disagree with that.[12] I think that it's crucial to recognize that people with very advanced dementia are still sentient human beings.

REFERENCES

1. Volicer L, Bloom-Charette L. *Enhancing Quality of Life in Advanced Dementia.* Philadelphia: Taylor & Francis, 1999.
2. Volicer L, Seltzer B, Rheaume Y, Karner J, Glennon M, Riley ME, Crino P. Eating difficulties in patients with probable dementia of the Alzheimer type. *J Geriatric Psychiatry Neurol* 1989;2(4):188–195.
3. Hurley AC, Volicer B, Mahoney MA, Volicer L. Palliative fever management in Alzheimer patients: Quality plus fiscal responsibility. *Adv Nurs Sci* 1993;16(1):21–32.
4. Fabiszewski KJ, Volicer B, Volicer L. Effect of antibiotic treatment on outcome of fevers in institutionalized Alzheimer patients. *JAMA* 1990;263:3168–3172.

5. Hurley A, Volicer BJ, Hanrahan PA, Houde S, Volicer L. Assessment of discomfort in advanced Alzheimer patients. *Res Nurs Health* 1992;15:369–377.
6. Mahoney EK, Hurley AC, Volicer L, Bell M, Gianotis P, Harsdhorn M, Lane P, Lesperance R, MacDonald S, Novakoff L, Rheaume Y, Timms R, Warden V. Development and testing of the resistiveness to care scale. *Res Nurs Health* 1999;22:27–38.
7. Drachman DA, Swearer JM, O'Donnell BF, Mitchell AL, Maloon A. The caretaker obstreperous-behavior rating assessment (COBRA) scale. *J Am Geriatrics Soc* 1992;40: 463–470.
8. Fried VA, Gillick MR, Lipsitz LA. Short-term functional outcomes of long-term care residents with pneumonia treated with and without hospital transfer. *J Am Geriatrics Soc* 1997;45:302–306.
9. Volicer L. Rheaume Y, Brown J, Fabiszewski K, Brady R. Hospice approach to the treatment of patients with advanced dementia of the Alzheimer type. *JAMA* 1986:256:2210–2213.
10. Hurley A, Bottino R, Volicer L. Nursing role in advance proxy planning for Alzheimer patients. *Caring*, August 1994, pp. 72–76.
11. Hurley AC, Mahoney MA, Volicer L. Comfort care in end-stage dementia: What to do after deciding to do no more. In: Olson E, Chichen ER, Libow LS, eds. *Controversies in Ethics in Long-Term Care*. New York: Springer Publishing, 1995, pp. 72–86.
12. Volicer L, Berman SA, Cipolloni PB, Mandell A. Persistent vegetative state in Alzheimer disease: Does it exist? *Arch Neurol* 1997;54:1382–1384.

Bright Eyes: A Sensory Stimulation Intervention for Patients with Advanced Dementia

An Interview with SCOTT A. TRUDEAU, MA, OTR/L

Edith Nourse Veterans Administration Hospital
Bedford, Massachusetts

Scott A. Trudeau, MA, OTR/L is clinical director for rehabilitation at Edith Nourse Rogers Veterans Administration Hospital in Bedford, Massachusetts. He is formerly a clinical educator at the Geriatric Research and Education Clinical Center (GRECC) at the hospital, which houses the special care and dementia unit. While at the GRECC, Mr. Trudeau initiated the Bright Eyes program, a sensory stimulation intervention with men and women suffering from advanced dementia, which has resulted in improvements in their functioning and connectedness with the world around them. Although sensory stimulation is part of the repertoire of many activities personnel who work with elderly, cognitively impaired people, the Bright Eyes intervention is distinct insofar as it is a well-thought-out, theoretically grounded, and empirically studied series of activities provided by a medical professional. Mr. Trudeau reported the results of his research about the effectiveness of this intervention in a recently published book edited by Ladislav Volicer and Lisa Bloom–Charette.[1] In the following interview with Anna L. Romer, EdD, Mr. Trudeau describes the process of developing and implementing the "Bright Eyes" program and the outcomes he uses to measure its effectiveness in enhancing quality of life for elderly individuals with advanced dementia.

ALR: *Can you first describe the unique aspects of the long-term care setting in which you work?*

Scott A. Trudeau: Although in theory, it may appear that at our hospital we have more resources and staffing for research through GRECC than found in many other long-term care institutions, the reality is that we have faced, and continue to face, budget shortfalls and staffing cuts, and we are not insulated from those by research-allocated budgets. The biggest difference between us and some of your more traditional dementia care centers is that the mindset is different. It's sort of the philosophical approach to being able to do the research. There's a level of investment among staff and a sense that we can make a difference in the quality of life for our patients, which brings with it a level of optimism that may not be present in a lot of places that care for people with advanced dementia.

I think there's sometimes a sense of futility in other rehab settings about treating elderly patients, let alone those with dementia. A lot of rehab professionals still say, "There's nothing we can do about it. They're not our population." Those attitudes just blow me away. Then you add a cognitive impairment and you lose all hope of rehab professionals being involved. My view is that these patients *do* have rehab potential and they do have rehab needs. It's just that we have to understand that they're dying eventually from this terminal illness. But that doesn't take away that there is potential and there is hope and there are needs.

ALR: *What led you to develop the Bright Eyes intervention?*

SAT: I developed the intervention after reading the work of M. Carol Bowlby,[2] who is an occupational therapist from Halifax, Nova Scotia. Actually, it represents a practical, clinical application of her work. She first described her work using sensory stimulation applied in a sensory hierarchy, which begins with stimulating the sense of smell, then kinesthetic/movement (gross motor activity), and then moves to stimulate, in turn, the sense of touch, vision, hearing, and finally taste. In her model, these senses are stimulated in this order for a reason.[2] The sense of smell is a very primitive sense. I mean, the neural path that goes from the olfactory nerve to the brain is fairly short and direct, so even someone with advanced dementia or even someone who is unconscious might still have access to that sensory pathway. Using smelling salts, for example, can rouse someone who has passed out. It's the same kind of effect that you can get using a less noxious olfactory/sensory cue; people with dementia become awakened, in a way, through smell.

ALR: *In a given session with dementia patients, do you go through stimulating each of the senses in this order?*

SAT: Correct.

ALR: *Who worked with you to develop this application of Ms. Bowlby's work?*

SAT: There was a bunch of students over the years that have had an impact on it. But pretty much it's been my baby.

ALR: *Why do you call the intervention "Bright Eyes"?*

SAT: It came about in the following way. I came to the Bedford VA about 5 years ago after having worked primarily in acute psychiatry for most of my career.

When I came to Bedford, I was actually hired as the clinical educator for occupational therapy, which meant I would coordinate student programming. The GRECC had some special monies for stipend support to occupational therapy students, but no student had ever been physically placed in the GRECC special care unit although these students had done things for GRECC as part of their education. So, when I came on as clinical educator, I was initially charged to spend three hours a week devoted to GRECC developing programming. GRECC had previously been cited by JCAHO [Joint Commission on Accreditation of Health Care Organizations] for not having enough activities. So I said, "I can do an activity! Let's figure out which one." I started by doing arts and crafts with the patients because I had worked in acute psychiatry and that's what we had done as a rehab activity with people who had psychiatric problems. I started doing these craft kinds of things and found out fairly quickly that the elderly patients with dementia were not responding that well to it. They weren't connecting at all with the activities. They would do it in sort of a perfunctory, hand-over-hand way, and sometimes they would carry out the activity, but mainly, they didn't get into it. Then I found the Carol Bowlby book and said, "Ah ha! The whole notion of making an impact on the sensory experience may be more fruitful. Let's see what we can do."

I began to structure my arts-and-crafts interventions around a particular theme and included other sensory experiences during the process. For instance, one fall I focused on apples for quite awhile in these activities. We were working on sanding and painting apple-shaped trivets and every time we met we would eat applesauce or apples or smell cinnamon, and we had stuff that was apple-y around. Compared to the intervention we are using now, it was more of a bombardment in terms of the sensory experience. At that time, I still thought that what I should be providing was purposeful activity and, bringing my own baggage to the table, what I thought was productive had to result in a product, of course. But the patients just didn't connect with the product at all. I eventually learned that you don't need the product. It's the process that really gets you the payoff in terms of an impact on social functioning and quality of life. In my experience, when patients with severe or advanced dementia are not involved in these kinds of activities, they are often lined up around the periphery of a room staring vacuously into space. There's very little interaction that gets initiated by them. So, as I began to fashion the arts-and-crafts group into a more purely sensory group, I realized that we're really targeting the vacuousness in these patients, their lack of connectedness. If we made an impact, the folks would have bright eyes, because a connection would be made. So we call the intervention "Bright Eyes".

ALR: *Is the goal of the program, then, to get people to become responsive?*

SAT: Again, this is an area that I have come to learn a lot about. My goal is what I call "engagement." Now, in the literature, engagement is fairly ill-defined, and it depends in which context you're considering engagement—social, physical, marital even. But, basically, the notion of engagement is that, through some form of responsiveness, verbal or physical, there is a connection made to something outside of one's self. Then, that person becomes engaged beyond his or her internal world. That may be displayed as simply as reaching for a cookie or turning and making eye contact or as dramatically as someone who's traditionally mute speaking in the group. We've had some very dramatic responses from people at times, which I liken to what was portrayed in the movie *Awakenings*, but those are few and far between. I don't want to overemphasize the positive ones! And that's what I've really had to come to terms with—that I don't measure my effectiveness by whether everyone's talking or everyone's saying "thank you" or everyone's becoming verbally or even physically involved. I measure my effectiveness by the little things that happen. For example, for the kinesthetic movement part of the sensory hierarchy, we might have a beanbag toss. Typically, what happens is that folks will throw the beanbag back and forth to the leader and they'll focus just on the leader. A lot of times we work with primitive reflexes to get people going, so if you throw the beanbag sort of towards their faces, they'll put their hands up as a reflexive action to defend against that. They may or may not catch the beanbag. Then you work on getting them to throw it. After doing this whole routine for a while, you sometimes see that they take the beanbag, stop, look at it, feel it, move it around in their hands a little, and then turn to the persons next to them and hand it to them. Well, when that happens, I get goosebumps, and I say to students, "Did you see that?!" Because these people don't go beyond themselves. Part of that is their response to being in an institution, I think, as well as the fact that the disease is such that people become very internally oriented.

> *I don't measure my effectiveness by whether everyone's talking or everyone's saying "thank you" or everyone's becoming verbally or even physically involved. I measure my effectiveness by the little things that happen.*

ALR: *At what stage of dementia disease do people benefit from this intervention?*

SAT: The target population for Bright Eyes is people with severe to advanced dementia, people who are often mute and possibly not ambulating, sometimes near the end of life. But the program has also been beneficial to people who are less severely impaired. People don't mind engaging in the process even if they're more alert and more interactive. A skilled group leader will titrate the level of intervention appropriate to the individual and will get a range of responses depending on the degree of dementia. So, if I'm handing out pictures of Mickey Mantle and Babe Ruth when they were young players, somebody may only visually track the picture in front of them whereas somebody else may be able to tell you they have met Babe Ruth, or they remember him playing in Boston, or whatever.

Although one of our original goals for this intervention was to slow functional impairment, that has been hard to track. In fact, I once met Carol Bowlby and mentioned that that was one of our goals, and she said she thought that was not where we would see the biggest impact. And she was right.

ALR: *Can you describe what happens in a Bright Eyes group session?*

SAT: Approximately ten people meet in a group for about 45 minutes. There is usually one group leader, although probably two would be ideal for a group of that size. When I am working without students, I lead the group alone; or two students may lead the group together; or one may join me to lead it. The students always say to me, "How do you get someone to smell something?" It's very directive. You just go in and say, "Here. Smell this. Catch this. Throw me that." For the most part, the goal is to really focus on sensory experience and to get whatever kind of responsiveness we can out of the individual during that sensory experience. It's a very parallel group, in which the leader interacts with a single patient, then another single patient, then another. Now that's not to say that you can't stimulate folks to pass the beanbag to one another, or actually throw the ball across the room, or, if we're using a balloon, once lofted, it will move around the room and around the group and people will become aware of one another in the group as a result of that. So, it's not always just a parallel group, but it's O.K. if it is just a parallel group.

One of the key things that I haven't belabored enough about the actual protocol is that, even though the sensory experiences are presented in isolation, they are connected by an overall theme, such as baseball. Today, students led the group and the theme was babies. For olfactory stimulation, they had baby lotion. They used pink and blue balloons for the balloon volley (the movement activity). For touch, they passed around a doll in a crocheted baby blanket. The students used black-and-white baby pictures of their parents or grandparents to stimulate the visual sense. They played an Olivia Newton John CD of lullabies for the auditory stimulation. I don't know what they did for taste today.

The reason why the concept of hierarchy works in terms of how this actually plays out is that there's a cumulative effect. When you take people who are just sitting there, vacuously drooling on themselves, and you have them smell something, and then you have them move and present them with sensory stimuli around the same theme, there's a cumulative effect. We have found that following this intervention, very frequently, when you bring around a silver tray of ginger snaps at the end of the group and present it to people who don't feed themselves, and you say, "Would you care for a cookie?" they say, "Thank you," or they look up at you and they reach up and take the cookies and eat them. So, that's where I think there's some functional payoff to the intervention, but I'm not sure how to measure it exactly or how to quantify it. I am currently designing a study in which I will use videotape recording to demonstrate the differences in level of engagement in the group that has the Bright Eyes intervention and in those not in the group.

ALR: *How do you choose who participates in the Bright Eyes group?*

SAT: It's pretty random; it's just whoever is up and available. For some people, it will be part of their treatment plans. For others who don't get up out of bed on an everyday basis, but who seem to benefit from the group, we schedule the time that they're out of bed so it coincides with when the group is being provided. So, the group composition is not completely random but, on a day-to-day basis, I tell the students to involve "whoever's there."

ALR: *How frequently does the group meet?*

SAT: Three days a week. But there's no reason why it couldn't be beneficial 7 days a week, aside from the fact that I'm just one person and there's 100 inpatients and about another 100 outpatients with whom we're involved. The group that meets regularly really only involves inpatients.

I've used the protocol in a couple of other ways. I've introduced it in a higher-functioning group in our adult day-care center and, because that's a group of people who are able to recognize a product, we might organize a cooking task that might include olfactory, tactile, and other sensory experiences integrated into the purposeful activity, which actually has a product as an outcome.

I've also used it to educate family caregivers who come to the hospital to visit patients and don't know what to do. If their loved ones are mute, but we know that they still have the reflex ability to catch a ball and throw it, we may suggest to a wife that she carry a Nerf™ ball in her pocket, so, when she's bored and she doesn't know what to do, and she's talked to everyone else in the room, and he doesn't seem to be responding to her, or she's not getting anything back, maybe it would be helpful to toss the ball with him for a while . . . and it would be good for her. We've had some just wonderful effects from that. Other people seem to respond better to music. For example, we would ask the wife when she comes for her visits, rather than just coming to visit, to bring her favorite tapes or his favorite tapes and to put them in a quiet area with a tape player so they can listen to some music. Or she might bring real family photos and sit with him and go through them. It can be very meaningful. It becomes more meaningful for the family caregiver in some ways. It makes the visit certainly a whole lot more pleasant for everybody.

ALR: *Have family members ever attended the Bright Eyes group and observed their loved ones being responsive?*

SAT: Yes. But, I'm not sure how I feel about it. One reason is that there's got to be a ceiling effect on the intervention. The group works for that one hour. But, if we did sensory stimulation with the group 24 hours a day, they probably would become saturated. And I don't know where that point is. So, one reason why I am ambivalent about family members attending the group is that at times, they have thought, "This is great. We need more! We need more! We need more!" Another drawback is that, sometimes observing the group leads family members to have unrealistic expectations and to feel hurt because the responses they observed in the group may not occur when they try to use the intervention themselves. "Well, he can do that, why can't he do this? He responded there, why isn't he doing it here? He did it for him, why isn't he doing it for me?" I've done it both ways and, at one point, thought it might be nice to include families, but now I prefer to do the intervention without family there. I found that having family present was far more disruptive to the process than supportive of it, which surprised me a little bit. For six or eight months, I chose to do the group during visiting hours because I thought it might be beneficial for family members to observe, but I no longer do so.

The other thing is that, as I said at the very beginning, my values that I brought to the table about what is productive activity are very different from what is meaningful to one's cognitively impaired elder. And I think that family members may experience a similar conflict of values; it's possible for a cognitively intact spouse to think that the intervention is demeaning because it's so low-level or so unproductive-looking. I think the staff had some conflicts with family because of that issue, too.

ALR: *Are there any other similar programs going on elsewhere that you know of?*

SAT: No, although there are a lot of people who say they do sensory stimulation with cognitively impaired people. Activity personnel working with this population come from a wide variety of backgrounds and perspectives. So, there's a range of approaches to sensory stimulation. I don't know of anyone else who's doing it quite this way.

ALR: *Are there any risks in using this kind of intervention with elderly people with dementia?*

SAT: This appears to be a simple, straightforward intervention, but it's very powerful. When you're dealing with peoples' neurological systems and sensory experiences and dealing with primitive reflexes, it's very easy for things not to go well, unless you're very sensitive to the cues and aware of the neurological impact of various interventions.

For example, if you use light touch instead of firm touch, you could very easily stimulate spastic muscle tone. So if you're trying to help somebody throw the ball, and you're not doing it firmly and effectively enough, you could actually cause more tone and make the person more uncomfortable and less able to throw the ball, really quite easily. It's a very fine line.

ALR: *What kind of impact might sensory stimulation have on people in the group who are in pain? Is there any possible negative impact to sensory stimulation for these patients?*

SAT: There's always that potential, especially when you can't get accurate reporting from the subjective perspective of the individual. So, you have to pick up on the cues. The way the protocol is written, it's designed to be a pleasant experience, and any time it's *not* a pleasant experience, for whatever reason, then either the intervention has to shift or the person is removed from the group.

ALR: *Have you studied the impact of this intervention on depression, which is common in people with Alzheimer's disease?*

SAT: I believe that behavioral interventions for depression can be as important as pharmacologic interventions, but we have not done any controlled studies of this.

ALR: *Are there any other barriers that you can identify to successfully implementing your approach?*

SAT: I've wondered whether there were a more cost-effective way to do this. I can't be everywhere. Can I train somebody to do it? I've been very reluctant to do that because, when I've tried to, it has been my experience that you can't teach people how to think like a certain professional. Whoever is leading the group needs to understand the neurological and musculoskeletal effects of the intervention. There are skills involved that aren't necessarily visible. Families sometimes don't recognize that there are skills embedded in the activity either.

ALR: *In terms of evidence for the impact of the program, can you give some examples?*

SAT: One of the most significant things that's happened, and it's not a specific patient response, is that when I came over and said I was going to do this, staff members who work directly with dementia patients told me, "You're crazy! You're not going to get demented people to engage in a group." And the reality is that, even though that was where we started, this group has been ongoing for $4^1/_2$ years now, and over time we have seen demented people engaging in the group more and more. It does work, it can work, and people here don't question it anymore. You can keep agitated, demented people engaged in the group for 45 minutes. You have to have some reason for them to stay, but you can do it.

ALR: *Is three times a week ideal? Have you ever tried it for more? Or would that be too much sensory stimulation for some people?*

SAT: My gut feeling, and it would really have to be tested, is that it could probably be beneficial on a daily basis. But three times a week has become sort of the happy medium. When I started it was once a week, then we moved it to two times a week, and three times a week has really become the gold standard for us. It feels like there's the potential for some carryover. One of the things that I typically do, more for the convenience of the group leader, is that I will focus on a theme for a whole week: Monday, Wednesday, and Friday. So if the theme is the beach, I may shuffle the cues a little bit, but I stay with beach-related stimuli; instead of touching the sand, you're going to touch a terrycloth beach towel, or rub oil on your hands, or whatever. Or I may use some of the same cues again, more for leader convenience than anything else, but it's possible that this holds a tighter context for people, it becomes a routine—and certainly routine is one of the strategies we use with cognitively impaired folks.

ALR: *Is there a time of day that it works best?*

SAT: Morning. Without a doubt. Everything works better in the morning. The group participants tend to be more open and available in the morning to experience what we want them to get. And that timeframe allows us to avoid conflicting with visiting hours.

ALR: *Has this program changed staff expectations about what is possible to achieve in terms of quality of life for people with severe advanced dementia?*

SAT: Yes. Now the expectation is that you *can* do things with folks in a group, and sometimes that's happening more and more. I'm no longer the only staff person here that would consider bringing a group of demented people together, whereas, when I started, I was the *only* one that would consider that! Staff members in recreation therapy and nursing, to some extent, now consider group activities for their patients with dementia.

This summer, our program is going to include all of the Bright Eyes sensory experiences, but we're going to try as much as we can to get people outside into the natural sensory world. Again, I'm not facing a lot of resistance now, whereas people used to say I was crazy.

REFERENCES

1. Trudeau SA. Bright Eyes: A structured sensory stimulation intervention. In: Volicer L, Bloom-Charette L, eds. *Enhancing the Quality of Life in Advanced Dementia.* Philadelphia: Taylor & Francis, 1999, pp. 93–106.
2. Bowlby MC. *Therapeutic Activities with Persons Disabled by Alzheimer's Disease and Related Disorders.* Gaithersburg, MD: Aspen Publishers, 1993.

Promoting Person-Centered Care for People with Advanced Dementia

An Interview with MARY T. MARSHALL

Dementia Services Development Center
University of Stirling
Stirling, Scotland

Mary T. Marshall, OBE, has worked to improve the care of older people for more than 25 years, as a social worker, lecturer, researcher and manager of voluntary organizations. In the following interview with Karen S. Heller, PhD, Ms. Marshall provides perspective on the care of people with advanced dementia from her vantage point as director of the Dementia Services Development Centre (DSDC) at the University of Stirling, Stirling, Scotland, an internationally renowned center for dementia research, training, and service development. The DSDC was one of the partner organizations in EACH (the European Alzheimer Clearing House), which was set up to identify and disseminate expertise and good practices in dementia care from throughout Europe.

Karen S. Heller: *What can you tell us about your organization's efforts to improve dementia care in Scotland?*

Mary T. Marshall: The Dementia Services Development Centre is an organization that exists to extend and improve services for people with dementia and their carers by providing information, training, research, and development consultancy. Although we do not operate directly with caregivers, the Centre provides advice, contacts, information, and consulting to any person or organization setting up or improving services.

The philosophy of the DSDC, reflected in all of our activities, is to promote more person-centered care of people with dementia. Person-centered care is based on the idea that, until recently, most people with dementia have been surrounded by a malignant social psychology, which damaged them as much or more than the actual brain damage. Changing those attitudes and the social built environment are two things that you can do a great deal

> *In most developed countries of the world, in which the population of elderly people has increased enormously in this century, dementia care is an area for which there are high and increasing demands, combined with fairly low levels of expertise, or only recently emerging expertise.*

about and, if you can get them right, you can really benefit people with dementia.

In most developed countries of the world, in which the population of elderly people has increased enormously in this century, dementia care is an area for which there are high and increasing demands, combined with fairly low levels of expertise, or only recently emerging expertise. Our Centre was started 10 years ago by a campaigning group called Scottish Action on Dementia to address this need for information, training, and sharing of expertise. When we started, we were the only such center. There are now six or eight organizations like us—one in Australia, one in Oslo, one in Dublin, and the rest elsewhere in the United Kingdom.

Although DSDC only serves Scotland, we became "European" when, in 1995, we partnered with the European project, EACH, which stands for the European Alzheimer Clearing House. EACH was started by a very eminent Belgian physician, Dr. Franz Baro, to be a resource of information and expertise for Europe. The organization was initially funded through some money for dementia research and information dissemination that was briefly made available under the public health policy directorship, DG5 [Directorship General 5] of the European Community. The EACH projects were incredibly diverse, including a focus on economic factors, ethical factors, and helping caregivers to sustain their care. Our Centre participated in some of the startup projects, including researching good practice in dementia care in European countries.[1]

Since 1997, when the EACH projects were completed, the whole dementia movement in Europe has become much more dynamic. There was a huge Alzheimer's Europe conference in London in July 1999, attended by more than 700 people. Alzheimer's Europe is now very well established and very energetic and has all kinds of projects.

KSH: *Where in Europe do you see the greatest improvements being made in the care of people with dementia?*

MTM: In Scandinavia. I think the investment in staff training, staff development, and new models is considerable in all the Scandinavian countries, and it's quite remarkable. For example, small domestic models of care, which are highly person-centered, are the norm in Sweden and increasingly the norm in Finland. I would also include Denmark and the Netherlands as areas where there are a lot of high-quality developments and constant improvement. I'm not saying it's all good. I've seen some rubbish, too, but it is remarkable what they're achieving.

KSH: *What accounts for their success?*

MTM: I think it must be investment. They're smallish countries, and they decide a priority and go for it. Finland and Sweden are fairly centralized, and if the central government decides it's going to happen, chances are that it will. So they have humane policies that start at the top and are energetically promoted.

In Finland, for example, the Center for Research and Development in Welfare and Health [acronym STAKES in Finnish], located in Helsinki, is a government research and development unit. That organization has done brilliant development work in dementia care. Annikki Korhonen, a really remarkable lady, is the civil servant who's been identified to develop dementia care in Finland.

This organization has applied the small, domestic-care model and has undertaken a whole set of other initiatives to make dementia care more person-centered. STAKES has very good day care, for example, and, ever increasingly, home care. The startling thing about Finland's experience is that it's all happened so quickly. Seven or eight years ago, that country favored a traditional big nursing home bulk-care model. But having decided to change it, the country moved fast.

KSH: *How would you compare progress in the British Isles and, in particular, Scotland to what Finland has been able to accomplish?*

MTM: The United Kingdom is a much bigger country, there's much less of a steer from the top, and far less investment. Nevertheless, I feel very optimistic about what's been achieved. I've been director of DSDC for 10 years, and the greater understanding of what can be achieved by improving the social and built environment is truly formidable. I think everyone now knows that the small domestic model is the right one, but whether they feel they can economically provide it is an issue. They can no longer say they don't know about it.

Also, there is a greater appreciation for what can be accomplished through person-centered care, in part because we and others have been hammering home the point for ten years, but, much more importantly, because people have been able to see what can be achieved with person-centered care. They can see people responding to highly individualized care in the way that they wouldn't have believed. If you start modifying the social and the built environment to tailor them to the individual you can sometimes actually see *re*-mentia, diminishing dementia. You can often see a leveling out of the deterioration.

> *. . . people have been able to see what can be achieved with person-centered care. They can see people responding to highly individualized care in the way that they wouldn't have believed. If you start modifying the social and the built environment to tailor them to the individual you can sometimes actually see re-mentia, diminishing dementia. You can often see a leveling out of the deterioration.*

There are still some totally dreadful services in Scotland, but I think even they are aware of the potential for change and are eager to achieve it. We've had a burgeoning of very big nursing homes, and some of those have dementia units, but the units are far too big. The standard unit size is 30 beds, generally in clusters of maybe three of those units. However, I think that even the biggest nursing home company these days would say it knows it ought to do 10-bed dementia units, it just doesn't feel able to do it. I don't think there's anyone defending 30-bed units for people with dementia. I don't want to tar them all with the same brush, however, because some of the private companies are providing the best small-scale clusters.

KSH: *What is the primary setting for dementia care in European countries?*

MTM: Although quite a lot of people have to be in some sort of institutional setting, the priority of all European countries is keeping people at home. There was a very interesting project based in the University of Glamorgan in Wales, called ETAS (European Transnational Alzheimer's Study), which looked at social and health policies in dementia throughout Europe and identified five themes, which applied to all European countries, and four, which applied to most. Keeping people at home and supporting carers to keep people at home were the top two themes in social and health policy related to dementia in every single European country. But the figures for the prevalence of dementia in Europe and the location of care are tricky because there's a very substantial number of people with dementia who haven't had a diagnosis.

There's no doubt that British policy is very clearly about keeping people at home. In reality, however, that hasn't been borne out in practice, because it's often cheaper to keep people in these large places. We've closed down a lot of our National Health Service long-stay provision, which has on the whole been replaced by private, for-profit nursing home care, rather than home care. But the momentum is in favor of home care.

KSH: *What kind of support is needed to provide good dementia care at home? And what kind of support do family caregivers tend to receive?*

MTM: It's hugely variable, because it depends on the carers' capacity and health, and the living environment. I'm very optimistic that some of the technologies that are increasingly available will lift the burden on carers a bit. If you get a package of home care, it can be all kinds of combinations. It could be day care five days a week, it might be home visiting or home respite service. In the United Kingdom it's a post code [zip code] lottery. It absolutely depends on where you live, because it depends fundamentally on the local authority (and the available skills, commitment, and budget), which organizes home-care packages.

In some areas that might mean properly-planned 24-hour care with a combination of health, social work, and voluntary and informal care by relatives and friends, packaged up into a fairly satisfactory mix of services. In other places, it might be a little bit of day care and the odd district nurse. It's very, very hard to generalize, and that, I think, is characteristic insofar as there is no minimum standard or national criteria for eligibility for anything. The same generalization could be made about provision of palliative care at home.

KSH: *Given the push to care for people with dementia at home, what provision is made to assist the family during the advanced and terminal stages of the disease?*

MTM: Most people die in hospital; it seems to have become a pattern. If you want someone to die at home, no one's going to object, they will support you. But that isn't the norm. In the United Kingdom, a family caring at home for someone who's in the terminal stages of dementia would receive help from a combination of health care providers, including the general practitioner, the home nursing service, the social work department, providing both equipment and staff, and what we call MacMillan Nurses, who provide short-term care for people who are dying at home. They are often used to provide pain management and overnight care, giving carers a break at night.

KSH: *To what extent is hospice care available for people with dementia in Britain?*

MTM: The interesting thing about the British hospice movement is that it is only now beginning to think about dementia. We at DSDC have been extending the hand of friendship to hospices for about three years. We have the impression that they occasionally had someone who's dying of cancer who did either have dementia or get dementia, but this was not a key issue. Up until now, hospices have overwhelmingly cared for people with cancer. But now the hospices are becoming more and more interested in dementia care, in part because there are more and more hospices, partly because they're managing people with cancer at home more effectively and partly because hospitals are managing these patients better. So, hospices are expanding their ideas of whom they can serve. I was invited, for example, to chair the hospice social workers' conference the year before last to stimulate some more thinking about dementia and, for the first time, one of my colleagues, who is our specialist in terminal dementia care, was asked to speak.

DSDC has done a literature review and key-actor interviews on terminal care and dementia. As a result of this work we got more money to develop a training course with our colleagues in Scottish hospices. The training consists of a five half-day course, which will start this autumn. If it's successful, we would hope both to repeat it and to turn it into training material to disseminate more widely.

KSH: *What about links between hospice or palliative care and dementia care in other European countries?*

MTM: There are ever increasingly satisfactory and mutually fruitful links being developed between people involved in dementia care and those in hospice or palliative care, but I don't know the extent of it in Europe. It didn't come up in the research we did for EACH. We didn't ask about end-of-life care specifically, but it also didn't come up spontaneously.

I suspect the reasons for this vary in different parts of Europe. I think the idea of dementia services is not well-developed in much of Europe. In Southern Europe, for example, it's still very much considered to be a family problem. The amount of input provided, both by the voluntary and the statutory sectors, is pretty small. In those regions they are beginning to awaken to the need to support family care, but it's still not well-developed.

KSH: *What needs to be done in European countries to ensure good end-of-life care for people with dementia?*

MTM: There are two assumptions that affect dementia care near the end of life. One is that poor quality of life is necessarily part of dementia, and the second is that people with dementia don't always need active palliative care. There are dangers in these attitudes.

A major barrier to good care near the end of life is the belief that because a proportion of the brain is not functioning, therefore feelings, both emotional and sensory, are not functioning; spirits are not functioning. There's an assumption, I think, of much greater levels of lack of awareness and lack of sensation than there's any evidence for. People with dementia, especially in the later stages, are often seen as some other species without normal feelings. So, staff caring for people with dementia may be unaware of or may not believe that dementia patients can benefit from all the important principles that we have in palliative care and the idea that there can be quality in end-of-life experiences.

> *A major barrier to good care near the end of life is the belief that because a proportion of the brain is not functioning, therefore feelings, both emotional and sensory, are not functioning; spirits are not functioning.*

Moreover, because people with dementia can't tell you that they're in pain, there's only very slowly beginning to be any interest in pain and dementia. There was a literature review on pain and dementia in the last edition of *The International Journal of Geriatric Psychiatry*, which didn't find a great deal of literature on this.[2] However, this article indicates that although pain management in people with dementia isn't always assessed or even considered, there is now a general raising of interest in the topic.

Based on our own small amount of research, our view is that there is a big need to counter the prevailing idea that people with dementia have no feelings of awareness of death or need for comfort and continuity. I think that a person-centered, more optimistic view of dementia care is still undiscovered in quite a lot of parts of Europe.

Our view is that where you get good dementia care, you get good palliative care because you get staff members who see the person as well as the illness. Sylvia Cox, a planning consultant here at our Centre, who has done some research in this area, believes that the one seems to follow the other—if staff are good at dementia care and person-centered care, then they're much more likely to have a sensitive and positive approach to palliative care. You also need to get people used to thinking that people with dementia need both health and social care working together.

KSH: *Does it work the other way as well? If an institution or staff are providing high quality palliative care in general, is it more likely that they would provide person-centered care to people with dementia?*

MTM: I think it would be less certain, because what you often get in places which haven't got a real grasp of dementia care is this assumption that these people's brains are shot. That their awareness and sensitivity and feelings are gone. I worked once in a truly appalling psychogeriatric unit where staff members used to say to me, "Isn't it just as well that the patients don't have any awareness of where they are and what's going on?" I think that is still an approach in quite a lot of places where the staff do not understand that people with dementia can feel to the end. And that awareness of death is not necessarily something that goes in a person with dementia.

I visited a day center for people with dementia in Australia where the main day-to-day subject of conversation was death. They knew they were dying and the organizer of the day center appreciated that they were preoccupied with that fact, so, she encouraged that kind of conversation. Her view was that in most places, staff members don't have that conversation with people with dementia because the staff can't cope with it.

I also visited a very good care housing unit in Norway, which faced a cemetery, and I asked, "Is that really a good idea?" and was told, "Yes, it stimulates really important conversations whenever there's a funeral." But I think that has more to do with the staff's ability to respond and not deflect that preoccupation than it is about the particular location.

Another interesting thing—and this is just an observation based on anecdote—is how often relatives will talk about moments of lucidity in their loved ones around the time of dying. There is a curious phenomenon in dementia. It seems that even the most disabled person can sometimes have a moment of absolute lucidity when the synapses sort of click. I've had numerous carers talk to me about that happening on the deathbed. I don't know that there's any hard evidence of that at all, but it is an interesting observation, isn't it? Astrid Norberg, a very eminent dementia expert in Sweden, has talked about how such moments undermine a lot of our preconceptions about dementia.

KSH: *Is there much advance care planning in the United Kingdom for people with dementia?*

MTM: It's very, very unusual in the United Kingdom to see tubes and drips in any facility caring for people with dementia, so I suspect that people are dying earlier. Certainly, we do get visits occasionally from people managing facilities in the United States, and they talk about a lot more interventionist treatment for very old people than we would expect to have here. Some people here do have advance directives, but that's very unusual and only in a small minority of the population. Generally speaking, people with dementia who had some kind of acute episode in a hospital ward would not have a radical intervention. My father, for example, got pneumonia and was allowed to die comfortably. Unless anyone had a very strong objection, I think that in general, people in such circumstances would be allowed to die. So, there wouldn't be a plan, as such, there would be an understanding with the physician.

Perhaps the more worrying side of that approach (which, I think is, on the whole, humane and proper) is that often assumptions are made about quality of life in people with dementia. "Oh they've got dementia, so we don't need to do X and Y." People might not get surgery they require, to remove a bowel obstruction, for example, simply because they have dementia. I get the impression from talking to some carers and staff in the field, that often patients with dementia in their care have a good quality of life and are actually quite enjoying themselves. Yet, if a person is hospitalized, the acute hospital sector makes assumptions that dementia equals poor quality of life and acts on that basis. I think that sort of discriminatory allocation of health service resources is a bit of a worry in Britain where the Health Service is under a huge strain in terms of resources. In a sense, that's more of a worry than our willingness to allow people to die comfortably before they've needed tubes and drips.

KSH: *In the United Kingdom, what efforts are being made to maintain connections and communication with people with advanced dementia?*

MTM: The big question is, when are people *not* able to communicate in some way or other? The skill that we have to learn is how to communicate with people who have lost verbal communication skills and not assume they can't communicate. In his novel *Scar Tissue*, which is clearly based on a real-life experience, Michael Ignatieff, who is Canadian, took the view that his mother, who had dementia, was still a whole person inside and the problem that he could not communicate was his, not hers.[3]

There has been an enormous burgeoning of interest in the United Kingdom in communication in dementia. We're moving very swiftly to a far greater understanding of the language of people with dementia, who often use metaphor and stories to share their views and fears. We have a research project, which is looking at a whole set of new skills in how you elicit the remaining language, and also how you interpret and facilitate nonverbal communication. I think that this type of research will have a major impact, once the skills are disseminated.

At DSDC, we've identified communication as one of the areas we want to specialize in and we now have two ongoing communication projects. Three or four years ago, we produced a substantial British text, called *Hearing the Voice of People with Dementia,* by Malcolm Goldsmith.[4] We've built a couple of projects on that. One is on using the arts to communicate. The other is on a whole set of techniques, including using pictures and typewriters, interpreting behavior, and discourse analysis. That links with very interesting developments in counseling people with dementia and psychotherapy in people with dementia. Some of our work is about people with dementia being more active participants in their care generally, commenting on it, making choices, having preferences. That's very current in the United Kingdom because we're aiming for a more consumer-focused model of service provision.

KSH: *Are you able to educate the family about this as well as staff?*

MTM: Yes. We produced a set of basic training materials for families. We're now in an exploratory phase, looking at a whole lot of new techniques. We're not alone. There is really a huge amount of interest in it throughout the United Kingdom.

KSH: *Please tell us about your project using the arts in communicating with people with dementia.*

MTM: We employ a poet, John Killick, who has spent the last five to six years as a writer-in-residence for a major nursing home company. He takes down the voices of people with dementia literally and edits what they say as poetry. His view is that people with dementia are natural poets, because they think in pictures and metaphors. He has now started to work with us, looking at a wider range of the arts. He is collecting information on existing projects, such as those that use dance and drama, and also initiating some very small projects in areas where he doesn't think there is work going on.

One of the new projects that he has set up is about giving cameras to people with dementia residing in a nursing home, seeing what they photograph, and seeing whether taking pictures is helpful to people in their efforts to communicate. He's also got a mime artist working in a nursing home to see if gesture is something that remains when other communication capacities go. So, there'll be a whole set of books arising out of that suite of small projects. He's writing up some of these projects now. Ultimately some training materials may be developed based on these projects, if there seem to be threads that run through that are useful to share.

Another colleague at DSDC, Kate Allen, is a clinical psychologist researching the effectiveness of a set of techniques to promote one-to-one communication and verbal communication with people with dementia. One technique she uses is to give someone a picture of someone else and say, "What do you think X thinks?" as a way of eliciting an opinion which the patient is not able to give you about him or herself. Another technique she is trying is using boards on which photographs and other images are placed, to which the person can point. This is a well-established communication technique with people with severe injuries who can't speak. She's also looking at discourse analysis and at interpreting behavior.

KSH: *Which health care professionals would be most likely to use these communication skills?*

MTM: They're mainly staff running units where people live, nurses and residential staff of care housing, long-stay hospital wards, nursing homes, [and] residential homes. There's also some work going on in a day center, but most of it is where people are providing 24-hour care.

KSH: *Is DSDC linked with any clinical settings officially?*

MTM: Not formally. But informally, constantly. Kate Allen is working in about ten settings, in which the staff are serving as action researchers. She trains the staff to identify patients or residents and to try different techniques with them. They then provide her with feedback. She's so closely involved, she's almost part of it. But she doesn't want to do the work with the residents herself, because she wants to know that ordinary staff can do it. She's a highly skilled, very experienced clinical psychologist, so what she can do is not replicable. We want techniques that are usable by front-line staff.

KSH: *Will these projects in any way inform the development of your palliative-care curriculum?*

MTM: Everything gets linked here. It's like a stew, because it's a very small group of people (twelve staff members) that know each other well and influence one another's thinking. We have a sister organization at the University of Stirling, called the Centre for Social Research on Dementia. We're very lucky in having very strong researchers alongside, who can undertake much bigger projects than we can.

KSH: *Any closing thoughts?*

MTM: I think the closing remarks are where you start from, which is that the two worlds of dementia care and end-of-life care have so much to offer each other. The exchange of ideas and closer collaboration will benefit both hugely.

REFERENCES

1. Marshall M. *Example of Good Practice in the Continuum of Care: A Report.* European Alzheimer Clearing House, 1998. [http://www.each.be/introduction/WP2/Good-Practices.htm]
2. Cook AK, Niven CA, Downs MG. Assessing the pain of people with cognitive impairment. *Int J Geriatric Psychiatry* 1999;14:421–425.
3. Ignatieff M. *Scar Tissue: A Novel.* London: Farrar Straus & Giroux, 1994.
4. Goldsmith M. *Hearing the Voice of People with Dementia.* London: Jessica Kingsley, Publishers, 1996.

Selected Bibliography

Part Five

Selected articles by contributors to this issue:

Hunt L, Marshall M, Rowlings C, eds. *Past Trauma in Late Life: European Perspectives on Therapeutic Work*. London: Jessica Kingsley Publishers, 1997.

Hurley AC, Bottino, R, Volicer L. Nursing role in advance proxy planning for Alzheimer patients. *CARING Magazine* 1994;13:72-76.

Hurley AC, Volicer BJ, Hanrahan PA, Houde S, Volicer L. Assessment of discomfort in advanced Alzheimer patients. *Res Nurs Health* 1992;15:369-377.

Judd S, Marshall M, Phippen P, eds. *Design for Dementia*. London: Hawker Publications, 1998.

Marshall M. *"I Can't Place This Place At All": Working with People with Dementia and Their Carers*. Birmingham, UK: Venture Press, 1996.

Marshall M, ed. *The State of Art in Dementia Care*. London: Centre for Policy on Aging, 1997.

Trudeau SA. Bright Eyes: A structured sensory stimulation intervention. In: Volicer L, Bloom-Charette L, eds. *Enhancing the Quality of Life in Advanced Dementia*. Philadelphia: Taylor & Francis. 1999, pp. 93-106.

Trudeau SA. Prevention of physical impairment in persons with advanced Alzheimer's disease. In: Volicer L, Bloom-Charette L, eds. *Enhancing the Quality of Life in Advanced Dementia*. Philadelphia: Taylor & Francis, 1999, pp. 80-90.

Volicer L. Goals of care in advanced dementia: Comfort, dignity, and psychological well-being. *Am J Alzheimer's Dis* 1997 (September/October):196-197.

Volicer L, Bloom-Charette L, eds. *Enhancing the Quality of Life in Advanced Dementia*. Philadelphia: Taylor & Francis, 1999.

Volicer L, Collard A, Hurley A, Bishop C, Kern D, Karon S. Impact of special care unit for patients with advanced Alzheimer's disease on patients' discomfort and costs. *J Am Geriatric Soc* 1994;42:597-603.

Volicer L, Hurley A, eds. *Hospice Care for Patients with Advanced Progressive Dementia*. New York: Springer Publishing, 1998.

Volicer L, Rheaume Y, Brown J, Fabiszewski K, Brady R. Hospice approach to the treatment of patients with advanced dementia of the Alzheimer type. *JAMA* 1986;256:2210-2213.

Volicer L, Rheaume Y, Riley ME, Karner J, Glennon M. Discontinuation of tube feeding in patients with dementia of the Alzheimer type. *Am J Alzheimer Care* 1990;5:22-25.

Selected family and patient perspectives:

Bayley J. *Elegy for Iris*. New York: St. Martin's Press, 1999.

Dyer J. *In a Tangled Wood: An Alzheimer's Journey*. Dallas: Southern Methodist University Press, 1996.

Friel-McGowin, D. *Living in the Labyrinth: A Personal Journey Through the Maze of Alzheimer's.* Thorndike, ME: Thorndike, 1994.

Ewing WA. *Tears in God's Bottle: Reflections on Alzheimer's Caregiving.* Tucson: White-Stone Circle Press, 1999.

Other selected citations:

Agency for Healthcare Policy and Research. *Clinical Practice Guideline, Recognition and Initial Assessment of Alzheimer's Disease and Related Dementias.* Guideline No. 19. [AHCPR Publication No. 97-R123] Rockville, MD: US Department of Health and Human Services, Public Health Service, Agency for Healthcare Policy and Research, September 1996. Web address: *www.ahcpr.gov* or *www.ahrq.gov*

Albert SM, Logsdon RG, eds. Assessment of quality of life in Alzheimer's disease. *J Mental Health Aging* 1999;5(1[Special Issue]).

Coon DW, Edgerly ES. The personal and social consequences of Alzheimer disease. *Genetic Testing* 1999;3(1):29–36.

Eccles M, Clarke J, Livingston M, Freemantle N, Mason J. North of England evidence based guidelines development project: Guideline for the primary care management of dementia. *Br Med J* 1998;317:802–808.

Eloniemi-Sulvaka U, Sivenius J, Sulkava R. Support program for demented patients and their carers: The role of dementia family care coordinator is crucial. In: Iqbal K, Swaab DF, Winblad B, Wisniewski HM, eds. *Alzheimer's Disease and Related Disorders.* New York: John Wiley & Sons, 1999, pp. 795–802.

Jennings B. A life greater than the sum of its sensations: Ethics, dementia, and the quality of life. *J Mental Health Aging* 1999;5(1):95–106.

Kovach C, ed. *Late Stage Dementia Care: Basic Guide.* Basingstoke, UK: Taylor & Francis, 1996.

Kuhn DR, Ortigara A, Farran CJ. A continuum of care in Alzheimer's Disease. *Adv Pract Nurs Q* 1997;2(4):15–21.

Lyman K. *Day In, Day Out with Alzheimer's Care: Stress in Caregiving Relationships.* Philadelphia: Temple University Press, 1993.

Maguire CP, Kirby M, Coen R, Coakley D, Lawlor BA, O'Neil D. Family members' attitudes toward telling the patient with Alzheimer's disease their diagnosis. *Br Med J* 1996;313:529–530.

Mahoney DF. A content analysis of an Alzheimer family caregivers virtual focus group. *Am J Alzheimer's Dis* 1998;13(6):309–316.

Mittleman MS, Ferris SH, Shulman E, Steinberg G, Levin B. A family intervention to delay nursing home placement of patients with Alzheimer's disease: A randomized controlled trial. *JAMA* 1996;276:1725–1731.

National Broadcasting Company. *Dateline NBC. Days to remember: Alzheimer's patients meet in writers' group to preserve memories and support one another* [transcript of broadcast, August 31, 1998]. New York: National Broadcasting Company/NBC News Transcripts, 1998.

Nelson JL, Nelson HL. *Alzheimer's: Answers to Hard Questions for Families.* New York: Main Street Books, 1997.

Post SG. *The Moral Challenge of Alzheimer's Disease.* Baltimore: The Johns Hopkins University Press, 1995.

Post SG, Whitehouse PJ. Fairhill guidelines on ethics of the care of people with Alzheimer's disease: A clinical summary. *J Am Geriatrics Soc* 1995;43: 1423–1429.

Small GW, Rabins P, Barry PP, Buckholtz NS, DeKosky ST, Ferris SH, Finkel SI, Gwyther LP, Khachaturian AS, Lebowitz BD, McRae TD, Morris JC, Oakley F, Schneider LS, Streim JE, Sunderland T, Teri, LA, Tune LE. Diagnosis and treatment of Alzheimer disease and related disorders: Consensus statement of the American Association for Geriatric Psychiatry, the Alzheimer's Association, and the American Geriatrics Society. *JAMA* 1997;278:1363–1371.

Solomon MZ, Jennings B. Palliative care for Alzheimer patients: Implications for institutions, caregivers, and families. In: Volicer L, Hurley AC, eds. *Hospice Care for Patients with Advanced Progressive Dementia.* New York: Springer Publishing, 1998, pp. 132–154.

Tappen RM, Williams C, Fishman S, Touhy T. Persistence of self in advanced Alzheimer's disease. *Image: J Nurs Scholarship* 1999;31(2):121–125.

Appendix A: Targeted Resources and Tools

Websites and pages within websites change addresses (URLs) frequently. We have included the name of the host organization and its home page so that if a link to a particular tool within the site no longer works, readers can navigate from the home page.

Part Two: Communication, Truth Telling, and Advance Care Planning
A. Tools from *Respecting Your Choices*™

The *Respecting Your Choices*™ *Training Manual* (1994, 1996) edited by Bernard J. Hammes, PhD, has been recently revised. It is now available as *Respecting Choices*™ *Advance Care Planning Facilitator's Manual* (2000) revised and rewritten by Bernard J. Hammes, PhD and Linda Briggs, RN, MS, MA.

To order a copy, contact:

Gundersen Lutheran Medical Foundation
Attn: Accounting
1836 South Avenue
La Crosse, WI 54601 USA
Phone: 608-791-4394 or 800-362-9567, ext. 6748
Fax: 608-791-4432
E-mail: labriggs@gundluth.org

B. Related Websites
The following is a targeted list of resources and tools focused specifically on advance directives. At the end we direct you to one physician-run organization in the United States that provides training in communication skills.

Source organization and home page	Specific document or tool
Aging With Dignity http://www.agingwithdignity.org	**Five Wishes:** A living will that includes personal, emotional and spiritual wishes of seriously ill persons; valid in 33 states and the District of Columbia.
American Bar Association Network http://www.abanet.org	**10 Legal Myths About Advance Medical Directives** by Charles Sabatino, JD http://www.abanet.org/elderly/myths.html
American Health Care Association http://www.ahca.org	**Consumer Information:** Several pages of definitions of commonly used terms, such as living wills, durable power of attorney for health care and answers to common questions about the use of these tools; see http://www.ahca.org/info/informat.htm

Source organization and home page	Specific document or tool
American Medical Association http://www.ama-assn.org/	**Shape Your Health Care Future with Health Care Advance Directives:** An online booklet produced and funded by the American Association of Retired Persons, the American Bar Association Commission on Legal Problems of the Elderly and the American Medical Association; see http://www.ama-assn.org/public/booklets/livgwill.htm
Choice in Dying http://www.choices.org/ New name: **Partnership for Caring, Inc.** http://www.partnershipforcaring.org/	**Choice In Dying:** the inventor of living wills in 1967, is a not-for-profit organization dedicated to fostering communication about complex end-of-life decisions. The www.choices.org/site offers a range of publications, including sample advance directives.
Health Care Financing Administration, US Department of Health and Human Services http://www.hcfa.gov	**Advance Directives:** A document that examines commonly asked questions about advance directives as well as providing key definitions and resources by state; see http://www.hcfa.gov/pubforms/advdir.htm

C. Patient-Physician Communication Training

The American Academy on Physician and Patient (AAPP) is committed to the improvement of communication, the doctor-patient relationship, and the practice of medicine through the promotion of teaching and research in medical interviewing and related clinical skills. AAPP offers faculty development courses for physicians and other health care professionals involved in training physicians.

American Academy on Physician and Patient (AAPP)
6728 Old McLean Village Drive
McLean, VA 22101-3906
Phone: 703-556-9222
Fax: 703-556-8729
E-mail: AAPPatient@degnon.org

Part Three: Moving Toward Family-Centered Care
A. Related Websites:

Source organization and home page	Specific document or tool
Supportive Care of the Dying: A Coalition for Compassionate Care http://www.careofdying.org	**Hints for Conducting Focus Groups:** A quick review of how and why to conduct focus groups; see http://www.careofdying.org/HOWTO.ASP

Source organization and home page	Specific document or tool
Edmonton Palliative Care Program http://www.palliative.org	**Resources for Patients and Families:** Several short pieces, including Frequently Asked Questions of the Terminally Ill and Their Families; see http://www.palliative.org/patient_family.html
The Institute for Family-Centered Care http://www.familycenteredcare.org	**A central resource for both family members and members of the health care field.** While primarily focused on pediatric and maternal-child projects, this site includes a variety of resources including Hospital Forum, a department with profiles of ongoing hospital-based efforts to promote family-centered care. A profile of the Dana-Farber/Partners Cancer Care Program which focuses on adult oncology can be found at http://www.familycenteredcare.org/dana-farber.html This institute also publishes a print newsletter entitled *Advances in Family-Centered Care.*
United Hospital Fund http://www.uhfnyc.org	**Publications page:** A source for summaries of recent UHF publications, including a special report entitled *Rough Crossings: Family Caregivers' Odysseys Through the Health Care System.* This report explores the transition into illness and caregiving and provides recommendations for change in the partnership between family caregivers and the health care system.

Part Four: Pain Management Near the End of Life
A. Tools and Resources from Anna and Stuart Du Pen:
Anna and Stuart Du Pen's website is located at http://www.PainConsult.com. This site provides resources, recent news and events pertaining to pain management for patients and providers.

Following are four additional tools from the Du Pen's Cancer Pain Algorithm.

Figure 7. The Cancer Pain Algorithm Progress Note

Figure 8. The Cancer Pain Algorithm Flow Sheet

Figure 9. Constipation Decision Tree

Figure 10. Oversedation Decision Tree

Pt. Name _____

☐ Telephone
☐ Clinic Visit
☐ Home Visit

Pain Assessment

Etiology Location

☐ New Site   ☐ Non–Cancer Pain   ☐ Etiology Unclear

☐ Consistent with known tumor sites   ☐ Treatment Related

Pain Location: _____

_____

Character	☐ Nociceptive	☐ Mixed	☐ Neuropathic
	Aching		Shooting
	Throbbing		Stabbing
	Cramping		Burning
	Tender		Sharp

Pattern   ☐ Constant   ☐ Episodic   ☐ Constant & Episodic

Intensity [0-10]

Site#1	Site#2	Site#3
____Worst	____Worst	____Worst
____Usual	____Usual	____Usual

Side effects

Nausea	☐ Y ☐ N	Dry Mouth	☐ Y ☐ N	GI Distress	☐ Y ☐ N
Drowsiness	☐ Y ☐ N			Constipation	☐ Y ☐ N
Delirium	☐ Y ☐ N			Myoclonus	☐ Y ☐ N

Drug Choice Decisions

☐ Pain Controlled   ☐ No Change in Therapy   ☐ Initiate S/E Protocol

☐ Pain Not Controlled   ☐ Maximize Co-Analgesics   ☐ Titrate Opioids

                            ☐ Sequential Opioid Trial

Reassessment

☐ Pain 0-3 Contact PRN

☐ Pain 4-6 Contact at least weekly   Next Contact Due _____

☐ Pain 7-10 Contact qd-q72h

☐ Side Effects Contact per Protocol

Notes/Plan _____

_____

_____

_____

Signature _____ Date _____

Figure 7.   The Cancer Pain Algorithm Progress Note

This tool is part of the Cancer Pain Algorithm, Copyright ©1999 Du Pen, Inc.
Reprinted here with permission from Anna and Stuart Du Pen.

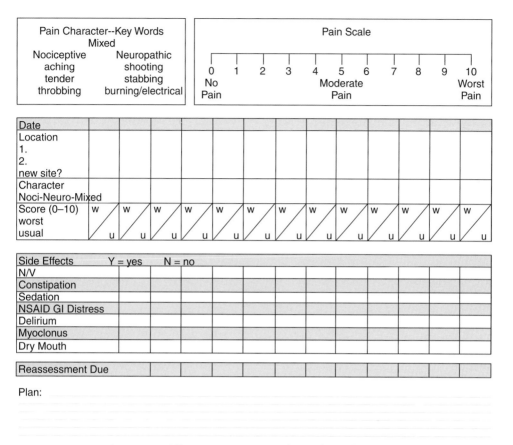

Figure 8.   The Cancer Pain Algorithm Flow Sheet

This tool is part of the Cancer Pain Algorithm, Copyright ©1999 Du Pen, Inc. Reprinted here with permission from Anna and Stuart Du Penn.

Constipation

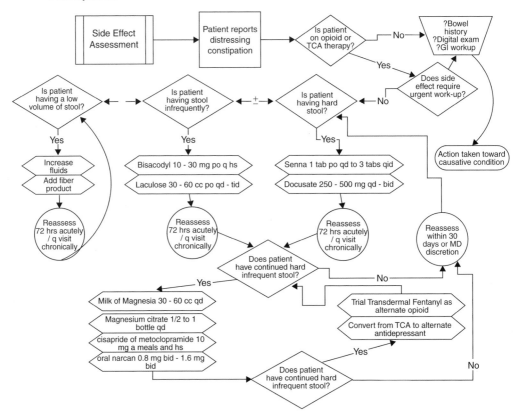

Figure 9.   Cancer Pain Algorithm Constipation Chart

This tool is part of the Cancer Pain Algorithm, Copyright ©1999 Du Pen, Inc.
Reprinted here with permission from Anna and Stuart Du Pen.

Oversedation

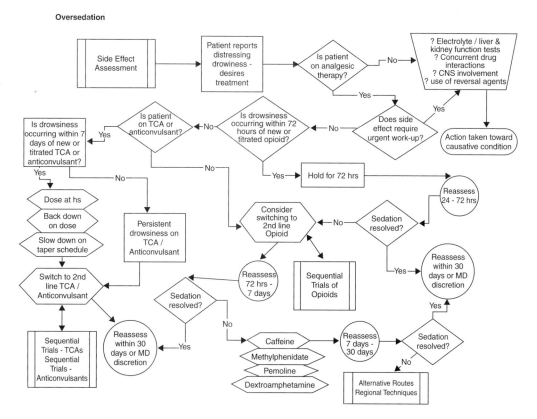

Figure 10.   Cancer Pain Algorithm Oversedation Chart

This tool is part of the Cancer Pain Algorithm, Copyright ©1999 Du Pen, Inc. Reprinted here with permission from Anna and Stuart Du Pen.

B. Related Websites

The following is a targeted list of resources and tools specifically focused on improving pain and symptom management for patients near the end of life. See PainLink at http://www.edc.org/PainLink/ for an annotated list of links to an extensive set of Web-based pain resources that are not limited to end-of-life care.

Source organization and home page	Specific document or tool
The American Alliance of Cancer Pain Initiatives http://www.aacpi.org/	**A Cancer Pain E-mail List Serve:** Hosted by the AACPI Resource Center. To learn more about the list serve visit http://www.wisc.edu/trc/list.htm
Association Internationale Ensemble contre la douleur http://www.sans-douleur.ch/ *Ensemble contre la douleur* is a francophone not-for-profit organization founded in 1997 in Geneva, Switzerland by leaders in pain management.	**Two Innovative Projects:** The site has updates from participating hospitals in the **Vers un hôpital sans douleur** (Toward a Pain Free Hospital) campaign. This campaign is not limited to end-of-life-pain, but *is a systematic effort to improve the treatment of* pain for all patients. Participating institutions are located in France, Spain, Belgium, Italy, Switzerland, Canada and the United States. A second major campaign sponsored by Ensemble contre la douleur is **Vivre avec le cancer sans douleur** (Living with Cancer without Pain). Additional information in French about both campaigns is accessible from the homepage. The site has a variety of resources including a bibliography with both French and English entries, a resource page providing links to French and English pain related websites at http://www.sans-douleur.ch/ai_fress.htm, and a French speaking list serve **sans-douleur** accessible from the homepage.
Cancer Pain Release http://www.medsch.wisc.edu/ WHOcancerpain	**Multilingual Specialist Newsletter:** *Cancer Pain Release* is published quarterly by the WHO Collaborating Center for Policy and Communications in Cancer Care at the University of Wisconsin-Madison. This publication is part of the World Health Organization global communications program to improve cancer pain control and palliative and supportive care. Some back issues are archived on the Web. French and Spanish versions are available. For more information contact the editor, Sophie Colleau, PhD, colleau@macc.wisc.edu; tel.: 608-263-0727.

Source organization and home page	Specific document or tool
International Association for the Study of Pain (IASP) http://www.halcyon.com/iasp/	**Pain Newsletter:** *Pain: Clinical Updates* is at http://www.halcyon.com/iasp/PCUOpen.html This site offers extensive links to other resources for dealing with pain at: http://www.halcyon.com/iasp/ressopen.html
The Joint Commission on Accreditation of Health Care Organizations (JCAHO) http://www.jcaho.org/	**New standards on pain assessment and management:** JCAHO won't be measuring compliance right away; visit their website to see the standards: http://www.jcaho.org/standard/pm_frm.html
PainLink http://www.edc.org/PainLink	**An extensive list of annotated links to pain related websites:** Visit http://www.edc.org/PainLink/plweb.html. *PainLink* is a virtual community of institutions and practitioners committed to improving their pain management practices developed by staff at the Center for Applied Ethics and Professional Practice at EDC in Newton, MA, originally funded by the Mayday Fund. The site has both public and members only sections. Members have access to a variety of resources including technical assistance, e-mail discussions, on-line events and the *PainLink* Clinician Survey.
Talaria: The Hypermedia Assistant for Cancer Pain Management http://www.talaria.org	**A hypermedia presentation of the AHCPR (Agency for Health Care Policy and Research) Clinical Practice Guideline, Number 9: Management of Cancer Pain:** Find this tool, as well as other multimedia instructional tools and technical information for treating pain at this site.

Part Five: Promoting Meaning in the Lives of Patients with Advanced Dementia
A. Tools and Websites Related to Contributors to this Part:

1. Film produced by the U.S. Department of Veterans Affairs:
Alzheimer's Disease: Natural Feeding Techniques
A 14-minute video that demonstrates how caregiving staff manage feeding difficulties for patients in the late stage of Alzheimer's. Includes three case studies that show how oral feeding techniques as opposed to tube feeding, can decrease infection, increase patient comfort and improve overall quality of life for the patient.

For more information contact:
Terra Nova Films
9848 S. Winchester Avenue
Chicago, IL 60643
Telephone: (800) 779-8491
Fax: (773) 881-3368
or visit their website at http://www.terranova.org

2. Dementia Services Development Centre
http://www.stir.ac.uk/dsdc
The Dementia Services Development Centre is part of the Applied Social
Science Department, Faculty of Human Sciences at the University of Stirling,
Stirling, Scotland. Its purpose is to assist in the development and
improvement of services for people with dementia and their carers. The
website lists publications and specialist reading lists in addition to pages on
development, management and training for healthcare professionals.

3. EACH: The European Alzheimer Clearing House
http://www.each.be/
The European Alzheimer Clearing House aims to bring together initiatives in
dementia care in the European Union in order to make better use of
existing information and expertise and to put forward and select examples
of good practice in the field of care for patients with Alzheimer Disease and
related disorders. This website is financed by the European Community and
offers a search engine and a wide variety of substantive information on
Alzheimer's disease and related dementias of interest to health care
professionals and researchers. This site offers many reports that can be
downloaded directly, including information on "Good Practice" at
http://www.each.be/introduction/WP2/GoodPractices.htm

B. Related Websites
The following brief list of resources and tools includes some targeted to
patients with dementia and their families and others to health care
professionals.

Source organization and home page	Specific document or tool
The Alzheimer's Association http://www.alz.org/	**Resources for persons suffering from Alzheimer's disease and their families:** The Alzheimer's Association is a not-for-profit organization devoted to education, advocacy and research on behalf of patients suffering from Alzheimer's disease and their families. The site includes a directory of more than 200 chapters across the United States and sections on the basic facts of the disease, caregiving issues, medical issues, research and news updates. Each section includes information directed to people suffering from Alzheimer's and their families as well as to health care professionals.

Source organization and home page	Specific document or tool
Alzheimer's Association NSW: Sharing Dementia Care http://www.alznsw.asn.au/default.htm	**Helpnotes:** Written resources for people diagnosed with dementia and their caregivers, some available in Chinese, Greek, Spanish and Polish; see http://www.alznsw.asn.au/library/libtoc.htm One noteworthy example is *Caring Tips from the Perspective of a Person with Dementia* by Christine Boden available at http://www.alznsw.asn.au/library/tips.htm Extensive international and Australian links are at http://www.alznsw.asn.au/links.htm
	Alzheimer's Association of New South Wales is an Australian not-for-profit community organization that provides support services to people with dementia and their families who live in New South Wales.
Alzheimer's.Com http://www.alzheimers.com/	**Offers a detailed overview of Alzheimer's management, treatment, risk factors, and prevention.** This site also includes other site reviews, resources, and links. A community message board allows patients and family to interact with others affected by this disease.
Alzheimer's Disease Education and Referral Center (ADEAR) http://www.alzheimers.org/	**The ADEAR Center:** A service of the National Institute on Aging, one of the National Institutes of Health under the United States Department of Health and Human Services. Visit the United States Federal Government Agencies: Resources on Dementia at http://www.alzheimers.org/federal.html
Alzheimer Europe http://www.alzheimer-europe.org/	**Guidelines for pursuing research and links to information about research projects co-financed by the European Commission in 1997:** Visit http://www.alzheimer-europe.org/ec97.html
	Specific set of tools for setting up an Alzheimer's telephone hotline: Visit http://www.alzheimer-europe.org/help_manual.html
	The site has information in English, French, Greek, Italian, Spanish, Dutch, Portuguese, Swedish, Danish and Finnish. Alzheimer Europe is a Non-Governmental Organization that aims to raise awareness of all forms of dementia.
Coping: Caregivers Helping Other Caregivers http://www.bhoffcomp.com.coping/	**This site is produced and maintained by the Men's Alzheimer Support Group of Rochester, Minnesota.** It provides extensive information on current medical news and information for patients, friends or relatives of patients diagnosed with Alzheimer's Disease and other forms of dementia.

Source organization and home page	*Specific document or tool*
Elder Books: The Alzheimer's Bookshelf http:/www.elderbooks.com/pages/about.htm	**A book publisher that specializes in books related toAlzheimer's disease.** The bookshelf page lists books and links to short descriptions and ordering information.
Mental Health Net http://mentalhelp.net/	The site provides an extensive list of annotated links to web resources that focus on Alzheimer's disease, dementia and geriatric resources. Visit http://mentalhelp.net/guide/aging.htm
Reach: Resources For Enhancing Alzheimer's Caregiver Health http://www.edc.gsph.pitt.edu/REACH/	**REACH is an initiative started in 1995 by the National Institutes of Health.** Its primary purpose is to develop and test new ways to help families manage the daily activities and the stresses of caring for people with Alzheimer's disease or related disorders. Progress reports on research projects supported by the National Institute on Aging and the National Institute of Nursing Research are at http://www.edc.gsph.pitt.edu/reach/progress.html and a bibliography of REACH related journal publications is at http://www.edc.gsph.pitt.edu/REACH/biblio.html
Time Slips http://www.timeslips.org/	**An interactive, intergenerational storytelling project created by a team of artists working with caregivers and people with Alzheimer's disease.** This site describes storytelling workshops that tap the creative expression of people with Alzheimer's and other dementias; includes sample stories by participants and has links to aging and arts related sites.
Undying Love http://www.rockymountainnews.com/undyinglove/	**A Personal Account:** Patrick Davison has created a photo essay and narrative account of his mother's life and experience with Alzheimer's disease.

Appendix B: End-of-Life Care Web Sites

Web sites based in countries other than the United States are listed first, followed by Web sites based in the United States

A. Web Sites Outside the United States:

Association Internationale Ensemble Contre la Douleur
http://www.sans-douleur.ch/

Ensemble Contre la Douleur is a francophone not-for-profit organization founded in 1997 in Geneva, Switzerland, by leaders in pain management. The site hosts information primarily in French and has information on its two campaigns: *Vers un hôpital sans douleur* (Toward a Pain Free Hospital) and *Vivre avec le cancer sans douleur* (Living with Cancer Without Pain). The site hosts a bibliography with both French and English entries as well as a resource page, providing links to French and English pain-related websites at http://www.sans-douleur.ch/ai-fress.htm and a French speaking list.serv *sans-douleur,* which is accessible from the home page.

Australasian Palliative Link International (APLI)
http://www.petermac.unimelb.edu.au/apli/

APLI is a group of palliative care personnel and supporters interested in the development of palliative care globally. The site provides a forum for the exchange of information, ideas, and initiatives of individuals and services and seeks to raise awareness of the needs of developing services and to formulate strategies for applying existing knowledge to local problems.

British Medical Journal
http://www.bmj.com

This site contains the full text of all articles published in the weekly *British Medical Journal* from January 1996. Access to the entire site is free.

Edmonton Palliative Care Program
http://www.palliative.org/

This is an extensive palliative care site for both professional and nonprofessional audiences, offered by the Division of Palliative Medicine, Department of Oncology, University of Alberta, Edmonton, Canada, and The Edmonton Regional Palliative Care Program. The purpose of the site is to acquaint the visitor with the basic philosophy of palliative care and its workings in large or small centers. Content includes clinical information, patient-assessment tools, cancer material, and links to related resources.

European Association for Palliative Care (EAPC)
http://www.eapcare.org

The EAPC was founded with 40 individual members in 1988. It is now a federation of national and regional societies of palliative care, representing more than 25,000 individuals across Europe and other parts of the world. The website serves as an information source about the EAPC and its activities, including descriptions of publications and congresses. The website also offers a directory of participating organizations around the world, including contact names and addresses. Many resources are available in French and English. A number of *Innovations'* editorial board members play leadership roles in this organization, including Stein Kaasa, MD, PhD, who is the incoming president.

European Journal of Palliative Care (EJPC)
http://www.ejpc.co.uk

European Journal of Palliative Care is the official journal of the European Association for Palliative Care, and is published six times per year. This website posts abstracts from the current and back issues of this print journal as well as offering an international calendar of palliative-care events.

Health on the Net Foundation
http://www.hon.ch/home.html

Health On the Net Foundation (HON) is a not-for-profit organization, headquartered in Geneva, Switzerland. The purpose of the Foundation is to advance the development and application of new information technologies, notably in the fields of health and medicine. The Health On the Net Code of Conduct (HONcode) has been created in response to concerns expressed to the Health On the Net Foundation regarding the varying quality of medical and health information currently available on the Web.

HELP: Helpful Essential Links to Palliative Care
http://www.dundee.ac.uk/MedEd/help/welcome.htm

This site is hosted by the Centre for Medical Education, University of Dundee, Scotland. Intended for an audience of medical professionals, this site has an emphasis on management of advanced cancer. Content includes pain management, management of distressing symptoms, communication issues, and emotional support for persons facing death and their loved ones.

National Council for Hospice and Specialist Palliative Care Service
http://www.hospice-spc-council.org.uk/indexf.htm

The Council is the representative and coordinating body for all people who are working in hospice and specialist palliative care in England, Wales, and Northern Ireland. The Web site provides information on a number of publications on hospice care intended both for the general public and for professional care providers, including a directory of all hospice services in the United Kingdom.

Sociedad Española de Cuidados Paliativos
http://www.secpal.com/

This is the website for the Spanish Association of Palliative Care; all content is in Spanish. Extensive information on the association as well a clinical guide to palliative care *Guias y Manuales: Cuidados Paliativos—Recomendaciones de la Sociedad Española de Cuidados Paliativos* is at http://www.secpal.com/guia.html and access to the journal *Medicina Paliativa* is also available at http://www. secpal.com/revista.html

University of Ottawa Institute of Palliative Care
http://www.pallcare.org/

The University of Ottawa Institute of Palliative Care is a Canadian academic center for research and advanced interdisciplinary education in hospice and palliative care. This site contains background information on the Institute and general information about Canadian palliative care and provides access to two newsletters (*Pall-Connect* and *News Brief*) for health care professionals. The site also includes an active conference area and discussion forum for the Canadian palliative care professionals.

B. Websites Based in the United States

American Academy of Hospice and Palliative Medicine (AAHPM)
http://www.aahpm.org/

This site provides an overview of the organization and its mission and information on events, activities, publications, and products of the AAHPM.

American Alliance of Cancer Pain Initiatives (AACPI)
http://www.aacpi.org/

As voluntary grassroots organizations, Cancer Pain Initiatives are composed of nurses, physicians, pharmacists, representatives of clinical-care facilities, higher education, and government. The AACPI facilitates communications and collaboration between initiatives, coordinates an annual national meeting, and acts as a national voice for the Cancer Pain Initiative movement.

American Association of Critical-Care Nurses (AACN)
http://www.aacn.org

The AACN is the world's largest specialty nursing organization with more than 68,000 members. Information about AACN is available at this Web site or by calling (800) 899-AACN.

American Association of Homes and Services for Aging (AAHSA)
http://www.aahsa.org/

The AAHSA represents not-for-profit organizations dedicated to providing high-quality health care, housing, and services to the nation's elderly. The Web site includes information on the organization and its resources and programs.

ABCD Exchange
http://www.abcd-caring.com/xchange.htm

Americans for Better Care of the Dying (ABCD), a not-for-profit public advocacy organization, publishes *ABCD Exchange*, a monthly newsletter in print and online. The newsletter offers timely overviews of end-of-life care issues.

American Health Care Association (AHCA)
http://www.ahca.org/

The AHCA is a federation of 50 state health organizations, together, representing nearly 12,000 not-for-profit and for-profit assisted-living, nursing facility, and subacute care providers that care for more than one million individuals who are elderly or who have disabilities nationally.

American Hospital Association (AHA)
http://www.aha.org/

The AHA is the national organization with close to 5000 institutional, 600 associate, and 40,000 personal members that represents and serves all types of hospitals, health care networks, and their patients and communities.

American Medical Directors Association
http://www.amda.com/

This is a national professional organization committed to the continuous improvement of the quality of patient care by providing education, advocacy, information, and professional development for medical directors and other physicians who practice in long-term care.

American Medical Student Association (AMSA)
http://www.amsa.org

The AMSA is a student-governed national organization with a membership of nearly 30,000 medical students, premedical students, interns, and residents from across the United States committed to representing the concerns of physicians-in-training. The Web site offers information on the organization.

American Pain Society
http://www.ampainsoc.org/

The mission of the American Pain Society is to serve people in pain by advancing research, education, treatment and professional practice. APS is a not-for-profit membership society and welcomes broad participation from all disciplines. Resources include the most recent information on public policy updates, reference tools, and advances in pain management.

American Society of Bioethics and Humanities (ABSH)
http://www.asbh.org/

The purpose of ASBH is to promote the exchange of ideas and foster multidisciplinary, interdisciplinary, and interprofessional scholarship, research, teaching, policy development, professional development, and collegiality among people engaged in all of the endeavors related to clinical and academic bioethics and the health-related humanities.

American Society of Law, Medicine, Ethics (ASLME)
http://www.aslme.org/

The mission of the ASLME is to provide high-quality scholarship, debate, and critical thought to the community of professionals at the intersection of law, health care, policy, and ethics.

The Association for Death Education and Counseling (ADEC)
http://www.adec.org

The ADEC, founded in 1976, is a multidisciplinary organization dedicated to improving the quality of death education, counseling and care giving; to promoting research; and to providing support, stimulation, and encouragement to its members and people who are studying and working in death-related fields.

Best Practice Network
http://best4health.org

The purpose of the Best Practice Network is to promote information sharing in health care by nurses, physicians, and other health care professionals. The site is a place where health care professionals can exchange ideas and share their collaborative best practice processes or systems.

Center for Applied Ethics and Professional Practice
Education Development Center, Inc.
http://www.edc.org/CAE/

The Center designs, implements, and evaluates solutions to health and community problems, accomplishing change in ways that respect the often conflicting values of a pluralistic society. A major current focus is on ensuring the wise and effective use of biomedical technologies and scientific knowledge to improve the quality of life and the health of the public. *Innovations in End-of-Life Care* is one of several current projects designed to improve terminal and palliative care.

Center for Bioethics, University of Minnesota
http://www.med.umn.edu/bioethics/

The mission of the University of Minnesota's Center for Bioethics is to advance and disseminate knowledge concerning ethical issues in health care and the life sciences. The Center conducts original interdisciplinary research, offers educational programs and courses, fosters public discussion and debate through community service activities, and assists in the formulation of public policy.

Center to Improve Care of the Dying (CICD)
http://www.gwu.edu/~cicd/

The CICD was founded in the belief that life under the shadow of death can be rewarding, comfortable, and meaningful for almost all persons—but achieving that goal requires real change in the care system. CICD is a unique inter-disciplinary team of committed individuals engaged in research, public advocacy, and education activities to improve the care of the dying and their families.

Choice in Dying
http://www.choices.org/

Choice in Dying, New York, New York, the inventor of living wills in 1967, is dedicated to fostering communication about complex end-of-life decisions. This not-for-profit organization provides advance directives, counsels patients and families, trains professionals, advocates for improved laws, and offers a range of publications and services.

Dying Well—Dr. Ira Byock's Web Site
http://www.dyingwell.com

On this site, Ira Byock, MD, past president of the American Academy of Hospice and Palliative Medicine, provides written resources and referrals for patients and families facing life-limiting illness and for their professional caregivers.

Growth House, Inc.
http://growthhouse.org/

This Web site is an international gateway to resources on life-threatening illness and end-of-life issues. The primary mission is to improve the quality of compassionate care for people who are dying, through public education about hospice and home care, palliative care, pain management, death with dignity, bereavement, and related end-of-life topics.

Hospice Foundation of America
http://www.hospicefoundation.org/

Hospice Foundation of America is the nation's largest charity. The organization's sole mission is to promote the hospice concept of care and which is supported primarily by individual nations.

Hospice Hands
http://hospice-cares.com/hands/hands.html

The purpose of this Web site is to promote the hospice philosophy by providing an interactive gathering place for the online hospice community, offering a comprehensive index of the hospice-related information available over the Internet, and adding to that body of information with original articles. The site includes an extensive list of links and articles and a chat forum.

Hospice and Palliative Nurses Association (HPNA)
http://www.hpna.org/index.htm

The HPNA is the only hospice and palliative nurses' professional association. Its purpose is to exchange information, experiences, and ideas; to promote understanding of the specialties of hospice and palliative nursing; and to study and promote hospice and palliative nursing research.

International Association for the Study of Pain (IASP)
http://www.halcyon.com/iasp/

The IASP is an international, multidisciplinary, not-for-profit professional association dedicated to furthering research on pain and improving the care of patients with pain. *Pain: Clinical Updates*, the IASP newsletter, is available at http://www.halcyon.com/iasp/pcuopen.html. The IASP home page also offers extensive links to other pain resources at http://www.halcyon.com/iasp/ressopen.html.

Last Acts
http://www.lastacts.org/

An initiative of The Robert Wood Johnson Foundation, Last Acts is a call-to-action campaign designed to improve care at the end of life. The goals of the campaign are to bring end-of-life care issues out in the open and to help individuals and organizations pursue the search for better ways to care for the dying.

Midwest Bioethics Center (MBC)
http://www.midbio.org

MBC is a community-based ethics center dedicated to its mission to integrate ethical considerations into health care decision making throughout communities. The Center offers workshops and educational programs for professionals and laypeople alike, assists health care providers throughout the United States in grappling with ethical issues in clinical work, and assists administrators in integrating ethics into organizational structures.

National Association for Home Care (NAHC)
http://www.nahc.org

NAHC is a trade association that represents the interests of more than 6000 home-care agencies, hospices, and home-care aide organizations. Its members are primarily corporations or other organizational entities in addition to state home-care associations, medical equipment suppliers, and schools.

National Hospice and Palliative Care Organization (NHPCO)
http://www.nho.org/
http://www.nhpco.org

Formerly the NHO, the National Hospice and Palliative Care Organization is dedicated to promoting and maintaining quality care for terminally ill persons and their families, and to making hospice an integral part of the U.S. health care system. More than 2400 hospices are Provider Members of NHPCO and more than 5000 hospice professionals and volunteers have joined NHPCO as members of the National Council of Hospice Professionals.

OncoLink
http://oncolink.upenn.edu/

This site offers a comprehensive guide to cancer information provided by the University of Pennsylvania Cancer Center. Designed for both professionals and patients, the site includes information on specific types of cancer, medical specialties, global resources, psychologic support, and information on personal experiences, clinical trials, conferences and meetings, prevention, and detection.

PainLink
http://www.edc.org/PainLink/

PainLink is a virtual community of institutions and practitioners committed to improving the pain-management practices developed by staff at the Center for Applied Ethics and Professional Practice at the Education Development Center, Inc., in Newton, Massachusetts, and originally funded by the Mayday Fund. The site has both public and members-only sections. An extensive annotated list of pain-related websites and resources are available to the public. Members have access to a variety of resources, including technical assistance, e-mail discussions, online events, and the PainLink Clinician Survey.

Palliative Medicine Program at the Medical College of Wisconsin
http://www.mcw.edu.pallmed

This site offers a variety of educational services and information for health care professionals about pain management and end-of-life care.

The Park Ridge Center for the Study of Health, Faith, and Ethics
http://www.prchfe.org/index.html

The Park Ridge Center is an independent, not-for-profit nonsectarian organization that conducts research, consultation, and educational programs on issues of health, faith, and ethics. The organization also publishes *The Bulletin*, a newsletter devoted to the connections between health, faith, and ethics.

Project on Death in America (PDIA)
http://www.soros.org/death

The mission of the PDIA is to understand and transform the culture and experience of dying and bereavement through initiatives in research, scholarship, the humanities, and the arts, and to foster innovations in the provision of care, public education, professional education, and public policy. The PDIA website provides a comprehensive overview of the PDIA Faculty Scholars Program, Grants Program, and Funding Initiatives.

Supportive Care of the Dying: A Coalition for Compassionate Care
http://www.careofdying.org/

The three priorities of the coalition are conducting research; developing models of comprehensive, community-based, supportive care for dying people; and creating a professional development program. The site has a variety of tools and resources and back issues of *Supportive Voice,* the newsletter of the coalition.

Dr. Joan Teno's Tool Kit of Instruments to Measure End of Life Care
http://www.chcr.brown.edu/pcoc/toolkit.htm

This site offers a bibliography of instruments to measure the quality of care and quality of life for dying patients and their families. Draft instruments are available at this site.

United Hospital Fund Hospital Palliative Care Initiative
http://www.uhfnyc.org/archive/clgrant/grpci.html

This initiative is designed to improve how New York City's hospitals care for patients near the end of life and for their families. The project has gathered extensive data about hospital deaths and is now developing, implementing, and testing a variety of approaches to improve care for dying patients in five hospitals.

University of Washington School of Medicine: Ethics in Medicine
http://eduserv.hscer.washington.edu/bioethics/

Ethics in Medicine is an electronic resource developed as part of the Bioethics Education Project, a collaborative effort within the University of Washington School of Medicine. The overall aim of this project is to expand and integrate bioethics education throughout the medical-school curriculum. The topics, cases, and resources covered are intended to be used as a resource by the University's community and to supplement or support other teaching and learning throughout the curriculum.

Veterans Administration Faculty Leaders Project for Improved Care at the End of Life
http://www.va.gov/oaa/flp/

The Veterans Administration Faculty Leaders Project is a 2-year initiative of the Office of Academic Affiliations, Department of Veterans Affairs, to develop benchmark curricula for end-of-life care and palliative care as well as strategies for their implementation and for training resident physicians. This project is supported by The Robert Wood Johnson Foundation.

World Health Organization (WHO) Programme on Cancer Control
http://who-pcc.iarc.fr/Publications.Publications.html

WHO publications, documents, and abstracts related to cancer pain, terminal illness, and palliative care are available at the site.

Contributors and Interviewees

Leslie J. Blackhall, MD, MTS, is the medical director of Assisted Home Hospice, Thousand Oaks, California, and a fellow at the Pacific Center for Health Policy and Ethics at the University of Southern California School of Medicine. She has studied Tibetan Medicine in India and in the United States and received her Masters of Theological Studies from the Harvard University Divinity School, where she studied cross-cultural and historical aspects of medical ethics. She is a nationally known expert on the care of dying patients and has spoken to physicians and other health professionals across the country on the practical, ethical, and spiritual aspects of death and dying. Her research includes a study of the attitudes of differing ethnic groups towards death and dying.

Thomas Cassirer, PhD, earned his doctorate in French literature from Yale University in New Haven, Connecticut and taught French and African Literature in French and English for many years at the University of Massachusetts at Amherst. While at the University of Massachusetts he and a colleague in Anthropology introduced a Five College interdisciplinary program in African Studies with faculty from Amherst College, Smith College, Mt. Holyoke and Hampshire Colleges. He retired from his formal teaching career in 1990 with the intention of exploring the concept of the Third Age of life, but he became increasingly preoccupied with difficulties in his marriage which he now understands were symptoms of his wife's growing affliction with Alzheimer's disease. In the process of reinventing a life with her, which he describes in his Personal Reflection in this volume, Professor Cassirer called upon a number of resources which have informed his understanding of love and education, including the example of his parents' 64-year marriage and his early education in two progressive schools, the Odenwaldschule in Germany and Bedales School in England. These experiences as well as his multilingual background, broadened by the example of African writers who had to have recourse to a foreign written language in order to express themselves, have contributed to his understanding of the predicament of a person suffering from Alzheimer's disease, and his search for a means of maintaining connection with someone who is losing her linguistic competence.

Anna Du Pen, ARNP, MN, is a masters-prepared oncology nurse with 18 years of experience in managing cancer-related pain. Ms. Du Pen earned her BS in Nursing, her Masters in Nursing, and her Nurse Practitioner Certificate from the University of Washington School of Nursing in Seattle. She worked with, and later married, Stuart Du Pen, MD, the developer of the Du Pen Epidural Catheter, and they are now referred to fondly around the country as "Du Pen and Du Pen." She has written many articles and book chapters on pain. Her areas of expertise include pain assessment, the use of an algorithm for pain management, and pain and symptom management at the end of life. Ms. Du Pen is a member of the American Pain Society, the International Association for the Study of Pain, and the Oncology Nursing Society. She currently represents the Oncology Nursing Society on the Provider Education Committee of the Last Acts Task Force, a multidisciplinary working group on end-of-life care sponsored by The Robert Wood Johnson Foundation. Ms. Du Pen is currently consulting for institutions around the country on the newly drafted Joint Commission on Accreditation of Health Care organizations' standards on pain management.

Stuart Du Pen, MD, is an anesthesiologist specializing in pain management, with more than 30 years of experience. His interests include management of neuropathic pain syndromes. He lectures widely on epidural analgesia and he is the principal investigator on two National Cancer Institute studies designed to enhance education of doctors and nurses about pain and improve pain outcomes. Dr. Du Pen earned his MD at the St. Louis University School of Medicine, and served as a clinical instructor for the University of Washington's department of anesthesiology for nearly two decades. He is the author of numerous articles and book chapters on pain management, and he is a member of the International Association for the Study of Pain, the American Pain Society, the American Society of Anesthesiologists, and the American Neuromodulation Society. In 1987, he developed the first Food and Drug Administration–approved long-term epidural catheter for cancer pain management. In the early 1990s, he and Ms. Du Pen (then a home-care nurse) had many heated discussions about selection criteria for the epidural catheter. The cancer pain algorithm was initially conceptualized as a template for ensuring that optimization of all conservative management was accomplished before interventional techniques were considered.

Stuart Farber, MD, is board certified in Family Practice, Geriatrics, and Hospice and Palliative Medicine, and has been involved in palliative care and hospice care for more than a decade. Four years ago, he left his private medical practice to pursue interests in medical education and research regarding end-of-life care. Currently, Dr. Farber is a Project on Death in America scholar and an assistant clinical professor in the department of family medicine, University of Washington School of Medicine, Seattle. Dr. Farber's current projects include a qualitative study of physician, patient, and caregiver perceptions of end-of-life care, within the Family Practice Residency Network affiliated with the University; initiating first- and second-year medical school courses in Hospice Training and Spirituality in Medicine; implementing a collaborative model for nurses, pharmacists, and physicians to manage patients with cancer pain at a regional medical center; and developing educational materials to assist patients and families deal with life-threatening and incurable illness.

Michael D. Fetters, MD, MPH, MA, is a family physician and assistant professor in the department of family medicine at the University of Michigan in Ann Arbor. He practices in both inpatient and outpatient settings. Bilingual in Japanese and English, Dr. Fetters directs the Japanese Family Health Program, an initiative that seeks to provide comprehensive, linguistically and culturally sensitive care to the Japanese-speaking population of southeast Michigan. Dr. Fetters has made multiple regional, national, and international presentations, and publishes his research in English and Japanese. Dr. Fetters attended Ohio State University College of Medicine, in Columbus, and completed his residency at the University of North Carolina Family Practice Residency Training Program in Chapel Hill, where he also served as chief resident. During his Robert Wood Johnson Clinical Scholars Fellowship training at the University of North Carolina, he earned a Master of Public Health degree from the University of North Carolina School of Public Health, department of epidemiology. He completed a Master of Arts degree with a concentration in anthropology and philosophy in the Inter-Disciplinary Program for Health and Humanities at Michigan State University, where he was a Lyle C. Roll Program for Humane Medical Care Fellow in medical ethics.

Shimon Glick, MD, is a native of New Jersey and a graduate of Downstate Medical Center in New York. He trained in internal medicine at Yale University Medical Center in New Haven, Connecticut and Mount Sinai Hospital in Bronx, New York. He subsequently was a research fellow in the laboratory of Berson and Yalow (Nobel Laureate) at the Bronx Veterans Administration Hospital, New York. Before his immigration to Israel in 1974, he was chief of medical services at the Coney Island Hospital in Brooklyn, New York, and clinical professor of medicine at Downstate Medical Center. He was president of the Association of Jewish Scientists, USA from 1965 to 1967. In 1974, he became professor of medicine and chairman of the division of medicine at the new Ben Gurion University Faculty of Health Sciences in Beer Sheva, Israel, where he was subsequently dean and head of Health Services in the Negev Region. He currently heads the Center for Medical Education and is a member of the Jakobovits Center for Jewish Medical Ethics at that school. He is a member of the Israel Ministry of Health National Advisory Committee on the Ethics of Human Experimentation and is one of the founders of the Israeli Society of Medical Ethics. He was formerly president of the Israel Endocrine Society and served as associate editor of the *Israel Journal of Medical Sciences.*

Bernard J. Hammes, PhD, was educated at the University of Notre Dame, receiving his BA in 1972 and his PhD in philosophy in 1978. He has taught at the University of Gonzaga in Spokane, Washington, and at the University of Wisconsin-La Crosse. Since 1984, he has served as director of medical humanities for the Gundersen Lutheran Medical Center in La Crosse, Wisconsin. In this position, he provides educational programs for the medical residents, medical students, and physician-assistant students. He also provides inservices and workshops for the medical staff, nursing staff, social workers, and the pastoral care department. Dr. Hammes chairs both the Institutional Review Board and Institutional Ethics Committee. For the Institutional Ethics Committee, he serves as an ethics consultant. Dr. Hammes' work has been primarily focused on improving care at the end of life. To this end, he has developed institutional policies and practices, staff education, and patient/community education with a special focus on advance-care planning. This work has resulted in two nationally recognized programs on advance care planning: *If I Only Knew . . .,* and *Respecting Your Choices.*™ He has authored or coauthored 12 articles and several book chapters that are focused on clinical ethics, advance care planning, and end-of-life issues.

Navah Harlow, MA, is director of the Center for Ethics in Medicine at Beth Israel Medical Center in New York City. She has created an ethics consultation service that provides support to both clinical and administrative staff as well as to patients and their caregivers. She conducts regular ethics rounds with medical staff members and organizes educational programming on a wide range of topics for staff members and the community. Ms. Harlow has been instrumental in creating hospital-wide policies and procedures for dealing with a variety of issues, such as access to ethics consultations, end-of-life issues, advance directives, and privacy and confidentiality in the electronic age. She recently served as principal investigator for a research project on palliative care, which resulted in the establishment of a department of pain medicine and palliative care at Beth Israel Medical Center. Ms. Harlow is a graduate of Boston University, magna cum laude, Phi Beta Kappa, and a recipient of a Masters degree in counseling from Columbia University, New York, New York. She has lectured widely both nationally and internationally.

Karen S. Heller, PhD, is a senior research and development associate in the Center for Applied Ethics and Professional Practice at EDC, where she currently directs two projects, Enhancing Family-Centered Care of Children Living with Life-Threatening Conditions and the national continuing medical education and quality-improvement program Decisions Near the End of Life. A medical anthropologist with extensive research experience in urban community and clinical settings, Dr. Heller has been a researcher in studies concerning end-of-life decision-making among cancer and AIDS patients from diverse ethnic backgrounds being treated at a large urban hospital; the management of chronic illness in frail elderly people living in the community; social interaction among patients and staff in a nursing home; and factors influencing whether HIV-infected adults seek early treatment intervention. She also has worked as a writer and editor and was formerly director of the Communications Office in the Division of Cancer Control, Dana-Farber Cancer Institute. Dr. Heller received her BA degree from Sarah Lawrence College, her MA from the University of Chicago, and her PhD from the University of California at San Francisco and Berkeley, and was a Post-Doctoral Research Scholar at the Stanford University Center for Biomedical Ethics, Stanford, California.

Ann Hurley, RN, DNSc, FAAN, CNA, is the associate director for education and program evaluation for the Geriatric Research and Education Clinical Center at the Edith Nourse Rogers Veterans Administration Hospital in Bedford, Massachusetts. She also serves as an adjunct professor of nursing at Northeastern University in Boston, Massachusetts, is a research associate at the Boston University School of Public Health, and an Education Core Leader at the Boston University Alzheimer Disease Center. Dr. Hurley is also a Colonel in the United States Army Reserve. She has published widely on many topics relating to Alzheimer's disease, with a particular focus on instrument development and palliative care management of persons with dementia as well as on promoting interdisciplinary grant writing. Dr. Hurley received both her Masters of Science and doctorate in Nursing Science from the Boston University School of Nursing. She has received a number of honors, including being named Distinguished Practitioner of Nursing by the National Academies of Practice and a Distinguished Nurse Researcher by the Massachusetts Nursing Association. She is also a fellow of the American Academy of Nursing.

Linda Kristjanson, PhD, is professor of palliative care nursing at Edith Cowan University, Perth, Australia, and director of hospice research for Silver Chain Hospice Service in Western Australia. She also serves as a research consultant to the Cancer Clinical Services Unit at Sir Charles Gairdner Hospital in Perth, Western Australia. Dr. Kristjanson leads a number of palliative care research teams, focusing on the care needs of terminally ill patients and their families.

Mary T. Marshall has worked with older people for more than 25 years, as a social worker, lecturer, researcher, and voluntary organization manager. She is now director of the Dementia Services Development Centre (DSDC), University of Stirling, Stirling, Scotland. The DSDC exists to extend and improve services for people with dementia and their carers. Previously, she directed Age Concern Scotland and was a member of the Royal Commission on long-term care for the elderly. She has written and edited several books about working with older people and about dementia care. Professor Marshall was awarded the OBE (Order of the British Empire) in the 1997 Honour's List.

Juan M. Núñez Olarte, MD, PhD, is a specialist in internal medicine and palliative medicine and is currently a practicing physician in the Palliative Care Unit, Hospital General Universitario Gregorio Marañón, Madrid, Spain. He has also worked in palliative care units in Canada and in the United States. He is a member of both the Board of Directors of the Spanish Association for Palliative Care and the Steering Committee of the Research Network of the European Association for Palliative Care. Dr. Núñez Olarte holds a PhD in History of Medicine and has published extensively.

Carla Ripamonti, MD, is an oncologist and clinical pharmacologist at the Pain Therapy and Palliative Care division of the National Cancer Institute in Milan, Italy, and is an adjunct clinical professor of oncology at Alberta University in Canada, where she is also a lecturer. Dr. Ripamonti's special area of interest is currently pharmacodynamics and pharmacokinetics of opioids. She is also a member of the Steering Committee of the Research Network of the European Association for Palliative Care.

Anna L. Romer, EdD, is a senior research associate at the Center for Applied Ethics and Professional Practice at EDC. A developmental psychologist and educator with a strong research background in medical education and physician development, Dr. Romer recently served on the steering committee for the National Task Force on End-of-Life Care in Managed Care and was a senior writer on its report, *Meeting the Challenge: Twelve Recommendations for Improving End-of-Life Care in Managed Care*. Currently, Dr. Romer is a coinvestigator on a study of family perspectives on end-of-life care at a Harvard-affiliated teaching hospital. She also has experience in writing, editing, and managing projects that are quite similar to *Innovations*. For example, from 1988 to 1990, she served as assistant editor of the *Harvard Education Letter*, a concise bimonthly publication that translates current research and theoretical advances into practice as well as spotlighting successful examples of reform in schools with the goal of advancing and sustaining innovative practice among educators. Dr. Romer is bilingual in French and English as well as conversant in Polish and has extensive experience living abroad. Dr. Romer received her BA degree from the University of Massachusetts at Amherst, her MAT from the School for International Training at the Experiment in International Living (now World Learning) in Brattleboro, Vermont, a CAS in Counseling and Consulting Psychology, and her EdD in Human Development and Psychology from the Harvard Graduate School of Education.

Mildred Z. Solomon, EdD, is Director of the Center for Applied Ethics and Professional Practice at EDC, where she has 20 years of experience researching, designing, and evaluating a wide variety of education and quality-improvement programs for health professionals, health care organizations, and the public. An expert in adult learning, professional development, and organizational change, Dr. Solomon cofounded the Decisions Near the End of Life program, which has helped more than 230 health care institutions across the United States improve practices and organizational policies to support the needs of dying patients and their families better. Dr. Solomon serves as Principal Investigator for Cancer Pain Relief in a Managed Care Setting, a $2 million researcher-initiated grant cofounder by the Agency for Health Care Policy and Research and the National Cancer Institute. She is also chair of the National Task Force on End-of-Life Care in Managed Care, which produced the report, *Meeting the Challenge: Twelve Recommendations for Improving End-of-Life Care in Managed Care*. Dr. Solomon received her BA degree from Smith College and her doctorate from Harvard University, Cambridge, Massachusetts.

Scott A. Trudeau, MA, OTR/L, has been at the Edith Nourse Rogers Memorial Veterans Hospital in Bedford, Massachusetts, since June of 1994, and currently serves as clinical director of rehabilitation there. Mr. Trudeau has filled many roles at the Bedford Veterans Administration, providing and developing occupational therapy clinical programs in both psychiatry and the Geriatric Research Education and Clinical Center. He has been instrumental in expanding occupational therapy student training and has conducted a variety of clinical research projects to explore the effects of occupational therapy interventions on the lived experience of persons with terminal dementia. Mr. Trudeau earned a Bachelor of Science degree in occupational therapy from Tufts University–Boston School of Occupational Therapy, where he graduated with honors in 1985. He returned to Tufts University, and in 1998, completed a Master of Arts degree in occupational therapy with a concentration on administration and research. In conjunction with this degree, Mr. Trudeau was awarded the Marjorie B. Greene Award for academic excellence and community leadership in May 1998.

Ladislav Volicer, MD, PhD, is the associate clinical director of the Geriatric Research and Education Clinical Center and medical director of the Dementia Special Care Unit, a 100-bed inpatient unit, at the Edith Nourse Rogers Veterans Administration Hospital in Bedford, Massachusetts. In addition, Dr. Volicer is a professor of pharmacology and psychiatry, assistant professor of medicine at the Boston University School of Medicine, and is a research psychiatrist at McLean Hospital in Belmont, Massachusetts. He is an external professor at the Third medical Faculty, Charles University in Prague, Czech Republic. Dr. Volicer has edited five books and published more than 170 papers on Alzheimer's disease, neuropharmacology, aging, and bioethics. He has served extensively as a reviewer of grants and has served on the editorial boards of three publications. Dr. Volicer received his MD from Charles University School of Medicine in Prague and his PhD from the Czechoslovak Academy of Sciences.

David E. Weissman, MD is a professor of internal medicine and director of the Medical College of Wisconsin Palliative Care Program. As director of the National Internal Medicine End-of-Life Residency Education Project, he is currently working to introduce end-of-life curriculum into 210 US internal medicine residency programs. Dr. Weissman co-directs EPERC, End-of-Life Physician Education Resource Center, a web-based resource for peer-reviewed physician education information, and he is editor-in-chief of *Journal of Palliative Medicine.*

Michael Zenz, MD, is a full professor of anaesthesiology and is the director of anaesthesiology, intensive care and pain therapy at BG University Clinic Bergmannsheil, Bochum, Germany. Dr. Zenz has published extensively on the treatment of pain and on pain policy. He has been chief editor for *Der Schmerz,* served on the editorial board for the *Journal of Pain and Symptom Management,* and worked as coeditor for *Current Opinion in Anaesthesiology.* Dr. Zenz is a member of the editorial board for *Innovations in End-of-Life Care.*

Zbigniew Zylicz, MD, PhD, was born in Poland in 1955. He graduated cum laude as a medical doctor in 1979 from the Gdansk University for Medical Sciences. In 1980, he moved to The Netherlands, where he was trained as an internist and oncologist at the Catholic University of Nijmegen. He holds a PhD in clinical pharmacology. Since 1994, Dr. Zylicz has been a medical director of Hospice Rozenheuvel in Rozendaal, The Netherlands, a pioneering palliative-care unit. He teaches palliative medicine at the University of Nijmegen, is the author of many articles and several books, and serves as a national contact point for The Netherlands within the European Association for Palliative Care.

Innovations in End-of-Life Care

Mildred Z. Solomon, EdD
Editor-in-Chief

Anna L. Romer, EdD
Associate Editor

Karen S. Heller, PhD
Associate Editor

Samantha Libby Sodickson, BA
Staff Editor

David E. Weissman, MD
Associate Editor

Editorial Board

A Last Acts Initiative
Supported by The Robert Wood Johnson Foundation

Index

A

ABCD Exchange newsletter, 204

Aborigine community, of Australia, communication issues with, 46

Access to services, 14

Acute care setting, transfer of dementia patient to, 155

Addiction, fear of, patient refusal of palliative care and, 134

Addressing of patient, sociolinguistics and, 95

Advance directives

  barriers to implementation, 26-27

  changing, 80

  as communication tool, 45-46

  with dementia, 156-157

  in determining patient's desire to know diagnosis, 96-97

  international approach, 13-17, 39-61

  legislation regarding, 29

  letter writing, intention of life support withdrawal, 69-70

    sample letter, 71

  Respecting Your Choices, 13, 20-37

  record, 37

Advanced dementia. *See* Dementia

African-Americans, attitude toward care of dying, 87-89

Aging with Dignity, advance directives resource, 189

Algorithm, Cancer Pain, 111-125

Alzheimer's Association, 198

  New South Wales, 199

Alzheimer's disease

  advance directives, 156-157

  advanced, 139-184

  Bright Eyes, sensory stimulation program, 165-173

  comfort, 159

  communication, use of arts, 183

  depression with, 159-160, 171

  mobility, 158-159

  patient perspective, awareness of, 153

  person-centered care, 175-184

  resistiveness in, 153-154

  spouse with, 145-150

  transfer to acute care setting, 155

  vegetative state, intermittent nature of, 162

Alzheimer's Disease: Natural Feeding Techniques, video, 197

Alzheimer's Disease Education and Referral Center, 199

Ambiguous disclosure, of cancer diagnosis, 94-95

American Academy of Hospice and Palliative Medicine, 203

American Academy on Physician and Patient, 190

American Alliance of Cancer Pain Initiatives, 196, 203

American Association of Critical-Care Nurses, 204

American Association of Homes and Services for Aging, 204

American Bar Association, advance directives, resource, 189

American Health Care Association, 204

  advance directives, resource, 189

American Hospital Association, 204

American Medical Association, advance directives, resource, 190

American Medical Directors Association, 204

American Medical Student Association, 205

American Pain Society, 205

American Society of Bioethics and Humanities, 205

American Society of Law, Medicine, Ethics, 205

Americans for Better Care of the Dying, 204

Antidepressants, use of with dementia, 159-160

Approaching Death: Improving Care at the End of Life, issuance of, 4

Ars Moriendi, 48-49

Assisted Home Hospice, California, 87-91

Association for Death Education and Counseling, 205

Association Internationale Ensemble Contre la Douleur, 196, 201

Australia, advance directives, 43-46

Australian Palliative Link International, 201

Autonomy, issues regarding, 15-16

B

Barriers to implementation, advance directives, 26-27

Ben Gurion University, Israel, 39-42

Bereavement in caregiver, 74-75

Bereavement support, 77

Best Practice Network, 205